CANCER ON FIVE DOLLARS A DAY

DOLLARS A DAY*

(*CHEMO NOT INCLUDED)

CANCER ON FIVE DOLLARS A DAY*

(*CHEMO NOT INCLUDED)

HOW HUMOR GOT ME THROUGH THE TOUGHEST JOURNEY OF MY LIFE

ROBERT SCHIMMEL

WITH ALAN EISENSTOCK

Da Capo
∞
LIFE
LONG

A MEMBER OF THE PERSEUS BOOKS GROUP

Designed by Linda Harper
Set in 12 point Adobe Garamond by the Perseus Books Group

Library of Congress Cataloging-in-Publication Data
Schimmel, Robert.
  Cancer on five dollars a day (chemo not included) : how humor got me through the toughest journey of my life / by Robert Schimmel with Alan Eisenstock.
     p. cm.
   ISBN 978-0-7382-1158-9
  1. Schimmel, Robert—Health. 2. Cancer—Patients—United States—Biography. 3. Cancer—Humor. I. Eisenstock, Alan. II. Title.

RC265.6.S29A3 2008
362.196'9940092—dc22

                                                                                    2007044913
All photographs courtesy Robert Schimmel.
First Da Capo Press edition 2008

Published by Da Capo Press
A Member of the Perseus Books Group
www.dacapopress.com

Da Capo Press books are available at special discounts for bulk purchases in the U.S. by corporations, institutions, and other organizations. For more information, please contact the Special Markets Department at the Perseus Books Group, 2300 Chestnut Street, Suite 200, Philadelphia, PA 19103, or call (800) 255–1514, or e-mail special.markets@perseusbooks.com.

10 9 8 7 6 5 4 3 2

Robert: for Derek
Alan: to B, J, K, and Z

This book is also dedicated to those who have fought the fight.
And to those of you that are just starting. Think positive.
Keep the faith. Find something to be thankful for each and every day.
And laugh. Take it from me, laughter is the best medicine.

CONTENTS

INTRODUCTION

I met Robert Schimmel in spring of 2000. Schimmel was riding high. He'd previously won the Stand-Up of the Year Award, his HBO special *Unprotected* was a huge hit, he was a frequent Howard Stern guest, and his Fox sitcom *Schimmel* had been picked up and was slated for a September start in the time slot following *The Simpsons*. Schimmel was white hot, somewhat surprising for a comic who was about to turn fifty, but long overdue to those who knew him. Schimmel was the comedian's comedian, the guy other comics would actually pay to see, the ultimate compliment because comics never pay for *anything*.

It was also surprising because Schimmel worked blue. *Deep* blue. He would often start his set without a hello and would instead begin by saying, "So this girl's giving me a blow job . . ." and he was off and running, segueing into a celebration of sex, a ninety-minute nonstop onslaught probing the pitfalls, frustrations, awkwardness, and sheer comedy that comes from coming. Was Schimmel ready for prime time? Or, more accurately, was prime time ready for Schimmel? Fox, known for taking chances and working close to the edge, apparently was unconcerned because the network had committed to thirteen episodes. *Emmy* magazine asked me to profile Robert, which I did for the June 2000 issue. Robert and I hit it off. After the article came out, we spoke for an hour on the phone and he invited me to attend his show at the El Rey Theater and the industry party in his honor afterwards.

And then it all came crashing down.

Schimmel was diagnosed with stage III non-Hodgkin's lymphoma. His chances of survival hinged on undergoing an immediate and aggressive course of chemotherapy. Robert informed his manager, the Fox executives, and the show's producers. The network put the sitcom on hiatus, which, in TV talk, means they dumped it. No sense investing in a show called *Schimmel* if Schimmel was about to die. So Robert lost his sitcom. And, of course, his fire went out.

But as his heat faded, he discovered something else. Something deeper.

When Robert Schimmel got cancer, he found himself.

Further, he came face-to-face with his soul. He saw that what he had been chasing his whole life up until then were mere *things,* material objects. Symbols of success and status. He realized that they didn't matter. A person's life is not defined by the size of one's house or bank account. Material things, Robert Schimmel realized, are immaterial.

Originally we called this book *I Licked the Big C—And I Beat Cancer* because during his chemotherapy, Robert never lost his sense of humor, his knifelike edge, and, most of all, his passion to entertain. At the core of Robert Schimmel's being is his absolute, basic need to make people laugh, even if the only people around him are suffering from cancer and the room he's playing is the Mayo Clinic infusion center. Going for the laugh is his survival mechanism, an instinct as primal as another person's need for food or water.

As soon as he was able to stay on his feet for an hour, Schimmel played Vegas. But he had changed. He refused to ignore his battle with cancer. In fact, he embraced it. He adjusted his act to include comic riffs about being diagnosed, smoking pot to alleviate his nausea, sex during chemotherapy, and losing all his hair, including his pubic hair.

But talking about cancer wasn't enough. Robert went way beyond that. He closed each set with a ten-minute Power-Point presentation featuring photographs taken during his chemotherapy. He punctuated each picture with a joke, but the underlying message was clear: my comedy is raw but my life is rawer.

Few comedians had ever revealed so much about themselves onstage. Here was Schimmel, emaciated, frail, hairless, at his most vulnerable—and his most powerful. For with this naked truth—this fearless depiction of his disease, his decision to share it publicly, and his daring to laugh at it—something rare, if not unique, was happening nightly between comedian and audience: a connection that broke all barriers. It resulted in both a creative release and an unspoken bond. I've experienced this before after certain extraordinary evenings in the theater. I'd never before experienced it in a comedy club. Schimmel would call himself a comedian; I would now call him an artist.

Interestingly, he wasn't less funny. If anything, he was funnier. This was measured by the sheer quantity and volume of the laughs. Before cancer, Schimmel was merely hysterically funny. After cancer, he nearly killed you. Every night when he finished his set and clicked off the last slide, the audience as one leapt to their feet. And as the house lights came up and the audience filed out of the club, their faces alternated between those who were still smiling and those who were overcome with tears.

One Thursday night in January at the Improv in Irvine, California, a young man named Jesse Gonzalez shared a table with his family. Jesse's brothers, sister, and mother had bought seventeen tickets to see Robert, Jesse's favorite comedian. The occasion was Jesse's twenty-fifth birthday— and the one-year anniversary of his father's death from cancer. Jesse and his dad had discovered Schimmel together a couple of years before during one of Robert's frequent appearances with Howard Stern.

Jesse remembered that first time. "Howard introduced him, then got out of the way and let Robert roll. He was amazing. At that moment my dad and I became his biggest fans."

That night in January, Robert had arrived late, just a few minutes before his set was to begin. In street clothes, his trademark suit in a plastic garment bag, Robert rushed into the men's restroom and changed for his show. Five minutes later, he strode down the center aisle of the club, applause rolling like a wave at his back, sweeping him onto the stage. Ninety minutes later, all pretenses at politeness had exploded.

The audience was on their feet, howling, clapping, five hundred strong delirious with joy and love, emotionally spent from both laughter and heartache.

Moments later, Robert, as usual, stood in the lobby signing autographs and selling CDs and DVDs. A line of people waited patiently to make their purchases, and possibly exchange a word, a handshake, and more often these days, a hug. Because Robert Schimmel, a newly crowned hyphenate—comedian/cancer survivor—now represented them, not only those who found sex funny and identified with Robert's raw and raucous take on life and love, but also those whose loved ones were battling cancer and those who were fighting or had survived cancer themselves. Robert spoke to them and for them. They waited to talk to him. They were in no rush. They would wait as long as it took to see him. And Robert, in turn, would wait for them, as long as it took to see them. He was in no rush either.

That Thursday, Jesse Gonzalez waited in the lobby with his girlfriend, his mom, and his older brother. Jesse was a big man, well over six feet tall and three hundred pounds. He wore a loose-fitting hooded sweatshirt atop a chocolate brown T-shirt that announced in sunny, happy-face script, "Boobies Make Me Smile."

As I stood to the side watching Robert interact with well-wishers, autograph seekers, and CD purchasers, I heard a soft moan. I turned and saw the big man, Jesse, begin to crumble. His knees buckled, and his brother and girlfriend grabbed him under his arms to keep him from falling. Jesse moaned again and started to sob. His face contorted in pain, he shook his head in a continuous windshield wiper motion. Somehow defying gravity, Jesse stayed in that position, hunched over, crying, clinging to his family, his arms draped over them as they held him up, for twenty minutes, until the line moved forward and he found himself facing Robert Schimmel.

Suddenly Jesse let go of his family and grabbed Robert with both of his meaty arms and held him in a body lock that fell somewhere between a bear hug and a boxer's clench. His body heaved as he continued to cry.

"It's okay, man," Robert whispered.

Two beefy security guards approached, prepared to step in between Robert and Jesse. Robert waved them away. They retreated, pressed themselves against the wall, a few feet away, just in case. Robert gently rubbed Jesse's back.

"I got you," he said.

To a stranger walking into the lobby at that moment, the tableau they made would appear ludicrous: an enormous man-child, his body towering above and folded over five-foot-six-inch Schimmel who, through the sheer strength of his heart, was holding up three-hundred-pound Jesse Gonzalez. Standing there, I knew that Robert Schimmel wouldn't let him go, that he would hold on to Jesse until he was strong enough to stand alone.

Robert had told me that at every show, people with cancer, friends and family of people with cancer, people who had lost loved ones to cancer, and cancer survivors would come up to him afterwards and tell him their stories. Sometimes they would just say thank-you—for his courage, his inspiration, and for making them laugh. And after each show, Robert would end up hugging strangers in the lobbies of comedy clubs across the country because even though they were strangers, they shared the same bond, they belonged to the same exclusive club.

Even though I'd heard about these moments, these instantaneous connections and spontaneous outbursts, I was unprepared for how emotional it felt. I saw how important Robert Schimmel, the man, was to someone like Jesse Gonzalez. I saw how approachable Robert was, how real, and how responsibly he reacted to Jesse's feelings. Other comedians I've known would have brushed him off. Seeing Robert hug Jesse and refuse to let him go, I knew that I was watching an act of extraordinary compassion, something that bordered on the *spiritual*, not the first word that comes to mind after a knockout comedy performance rooted in sex. I know now that in every Robert Schimmel audience there is always at least one Jesse Gonzalez and that Robert will always hold him up.

You can say that cancer gave Robert Schimmel more material. That would be true. But it also gave him more heart. The disease made him see the world through wider, wiser eyes. He became more patient, more resolute, and more conscious of the power of the moment. Cancer stirred him up and awakened him. And cancer taught him how to love what he *has*—his wife, children, parents, brother, sister, friends, and his gift, making people laugh; to love every day he's alive. His cancer story is a love story.

"My dad died of cancer," Jesse Gonzalez told me. "That destroyed me. I really thought I couldn't go on. When I heard that Robert was coming to the Improv, I had to see him. I had to talk to him. So I e-mailed him. He answered me. I couldn't believe it. He wasn't too good for me, you know? And when I saw him after the show, he hugged me and held me and told me that I had to live my life, but that I could talk to him or e-mail him anytime. I know that if he can get through cancer, then I can make it, too. He's a walking miracle. He saved my life. I love the guy."

That's why I'm writing this love story with Robert.

For Jesse. And Jesse's dad.

And for everyone who has been tapped on the shoulder by the Big C and told they were *it*.

Alan Eisenstock

CANCER ON FIVE DOLLARS A DAY*

(*CHEMO NOT INCLUDED)

SESSION ONE

"GETTING THE NEWS"

MONDAY MORNING, JUNE 5, 2000

So I'm sitting in a chair in my room at the Mayo Clinic waiting for the results.

I yawn and scratch my beard. I feel so spacey and hung over from the anesthetic they gave me. I think the guy went a little crazy on me. He was squeezing that IV in my arm like he was pumping up a tire. I check the room. There's my mom, sitting across from me, her legs folded at the ankles as if she's waiting for a bus. There's my dad, staring out the window, hands clasped behind his back. Contemplating the desert. Or wondering if my insurance is picking up the tab for the private room. And there's Vicki, my wife, sitting on the bed, flipping through a magazine. She's actually my ex. Well. Sort of. Kind of. It's complicated. I'll explain later because thinking about it now is starting to give me a migraine, which would really be the cherry on top of this sundae.

Nobody says a word. The room smells like ammonia with a hint of pine. And it's as cold as an igloo. At least it feels that way to me. You couldn't tell by my dad, who's wearing a short-sleeve shirt. I'm *freezing*. My teeth start chattering. A whole mountain range of goose bumps appears up and down my legs.

And this stupid hospital gown is riding up my ass. I try to pull it down and it snaps right back up like a window shade. I cross my legs and suddenly I'm Sharon Stone. Vicki sees this and rolls her eyes. Yeah, right. Like I'm flashing her in front of my parents.

"You're hanging out all over," Vicki says.

"What, you don't think my mom has seen me naked?"

"At fifty?" Vicki says.

She has a point. I cover myself as best as I can. Then I yawn, close my eyes, and shiver.

And suddenly, impossibly, I'm *above* them. Looking down on them. Hovering overhead like a bird. This is nuts. I must be dreaming. I'm either dreaming or I'm dead. Can they hear me? Wait a minute. There I am. Still sitting in that chair. I *am* dead.

Ma! Dad! Hello? Hello.

They really can't hear me. My mom uncrosses her ankles and sighs. My dad keeps staring out the window, then looks at his watch. Vicki tosses the magazine onto the bed.

I can't be dead. Okay, I wasn't feeling great so I went in for some tests and . . . *I died?* How did that happen? A thousand questions slam into my head, one after another, machine-gunned through my brain—

When did I die? Where is my spirit gonna go? Do I even have a spirit? Is there a God? What about Jesus? How does he fit in? I didn't believe in him on earth so is he gonna be pissed at me now? Maybe not because, after all, he is Jesus. What about my kids? Where are they gonna go? Did I ever finish my will? Who's gonna talk at my funeral? I'm not really close with any rabbis. I probably should've gotten close with some rabbi so I don't get the generic funeral eulogy. I hate those. You know he never knows the dead guy. He could be talking about anyone. *Robert was so special, such a good son, he will be missed. That'll be twelve hundred dollars.*

Below me, my mom looks past Vicki at a large basket of muffins, untouched, a bouquet of ribbons attached to the handle, the contents still encased in plastic. "Who sent these?"

"Fox," Vicki says.

"Mrs. Beasley's muffins," my mom says. She nods in approval. "Very classy."

"I love the lemon poppy seed ones," Vicki says.

"The minis?"

"Yeah."

"The best," my mom says. "Take a couple."

"Really? You think Robert would mind?"

"He's in a coma. You think he's gonna wake up and say, 'Hey, two of my lemon poppy seed muffins are missing. I go into a coma for a couple of hours and you steal my muffins?' Vicki, please, take a muffin."

Vicki shrugs and rips into the plastic muffin wrap.

"We never had a catch," my dad suddenly says, his eyes still peering out the window.

"What?" my mom says. "What are you mumbling?"

"Me, Robert. We never played ball."

"Sure, you did. Plenty of times."

"That was Jeff. Robert was too busy tinkering with his trains. Playing pretend games. Looking at girlie magazines."

He grunts, eyes still focused on something far away. "I have regrets. We never went fishing, hunting, none of those things."

My mom stares at him. "What hunting and fishing? We're Jewish."

Vicki, cheeks wide as a chipmunk's, stares at me propped up in the chair. "Look at him," she says, through a mouthful of muffins. "So pathetic. So sad. You know, Robert told me many times he didn't want to go like this."

My mother squints at her. "What do you mean?"

"Like this. A vegetable." Vicki swallows the last of her muffin, then with her pinky pokes at a poppy seed jammed between her teeth. "I think we should pull the plug."

No! I scream, still aloft, fluttering above them, desperate, helpless. *I'm right up here! Look! Help!*

"Otto, what do you think?" my mother says. "Should we unplug him? It's getting late. We leave now, we beat the traffic."

"We never restored a car together," my father says. "Never went camping. Built a doghouse—"

"If we pull the plug, we have to divvy up the muffins. I insist," says Vicki.

"I only like the lemon poppy seed and you ate all of those," my mother says.

STOP! I scream.

And then my legs feel heavy, immense, as if they're made of iron, and suddenly I plummet downward like a shot and I'm—

In my bed. Blinking. My mom and dad sit across from me. Vicki isn't here. There are no muffins. I remember now. My dad brought me in. My mom came later. She called Vicki, told her what happened, and said she'd let her know when we had the results.

"Wow," I say.

"You were out," my dad says.

"I had some dream." I sit up slowly, rub my eyes. "Has the doctor been in?"

"Not yet," my mom says.

"Wow," I say again, and then I laugh. "That was nuts. This whole thing has been nuts."

My mother shifts in her chair. My dad dips his head, studies his hands. There is dread etched into their faces. These are two people who have survived the Holocaust and then the loss of their grandson, Vicki's and my son Derek. They have endured more than their share of bad news and days of horror.

"Am I rich and famous yet?" I say.

My dad cracks a smile. "Not yet."

"Who's gonna play me in your show?" my mom asks.

"Meryl Streep," I say.

"She doesn't look like me. Plus she chews the scenery."

"Ma, we talked about this. You might not even be in the show."

She shrugs. "Fine. So it won't be any good."

Now I smile and try to piece together what's happened over the last couple of weeks, during the shooting of my sitcom pilot, then performing in Vegas, and the events come rushing at me at warp speed with the force of a tornado blowing through a pile of leaves—

• • • • •

I am in Los Angeles. I am separated from Vicki and living with Melissa. More about her in a bit. As soon as the pilot is finished and I get everything straightened out, I'll settle in L.A. for good, with Melissa.

Vicki and I have had a checkered relationship. We got married, then got the marriage annulled, then got remarried, got divorced, then remarried, then on the way to divorce for the absolute final time, no turning back, no bullshit, Derek got sick. We stayed together for him, for our other kids, fought the good fight, lost, then drifted apart, not uncommon when a couple loses a child. Now, unfortunately but inevitably, it's over, the final divorce. Bottom line, we tried. But it wasn't meant to be.

And now Melissa. Finding her, falling in love with her, realizing that I belong with her, being more certain of that than of anything in my life. And then, wham, there's a light shining on me, as if the spotlight finds me for the first time. I'm asked to do a sitcom. Me? You kidding? I'm fifty, bald, and Jewish. Not exactly the demographic advertisers are trying to reel in. Who cares? It's my time. After twenty years of stand-up, America has embraced me and my raw, take-no-prisoners, balls-out comedy. I'm gonna be famous. Bizarre.

I go into rehearsal for the pilot. The hours are grueling, the work is intense. I feel fatigued and dazed, and then right before we're set to shoot the show, I start getting chills, two, three times a night. I've got the shakes so bad that I pile on extra blankets. When I wake up, the bed is soaked, totally drenched, as if a pipe has burst beneath the sheets. Melissa is worried, begs me to see a doctor. I don't know any doctors in L.A. I call my manager, who makes an appointment for me with his doctor. I go in for a checkup, and the doc schedules me for a CAT scan. The scan comes back clean.

"You're run down," the doctor says. "We might want to do more tests. You could have Epstein-Barr or mono. That'd be my guess."

Even though there's nothing on the scan, something eats at me. I don't know why, but I feel like there's something else, something that the scan didn't see.

About a week after we shoot the pilot, I'm playing the Monte Carlo in Vegas. My parents are staying with me. It's early June and by noon the temperature is hitting 110, but no problem, it's a dry heat. One afternoon, my dad and I decide to take a stroll through the forum shops. Suddenly, I'm freezing. My entire body starts to shiver. My lips quiver and my teeth begin to chatter.

"Robert, you're shaking."

"I'm freezing. I'm gonna go into the Gap and buy a sweatshirt. I'm really cold."

"Have you seen a doctor?"

"Yeah. I saw that guy in L.A."

"You have to get a second opinion. Today."

I call the doctor who removed my gall bladder a few years ago. He sets me up the next day with a doctor at Mayo in Scottsdale. The doctor wears a permanent frown as he goes over me like he's buying a used car. Finally he says, "How long have you had this lump?"

"Lump? Where?"

"Right here." He lifts my left arm and rubs a tiny bump in my armpit, half the size of a pea.

"I didn't know I had that."

The doctor puckers his lips. For a second it looks like he's gonna kiss me. Then he whistles out a thin stream of air.

"Feels funny," he says. "I want to do a biopsy."

And that's how I ended up here at the Mayo Clinic, my parents sitting bedside, nobody saying much. All of us waiting for the news.

Actually, there's another curve ball. When I woke up in the recovery room, after some of the anesthetic wore off, I felt pain shooting up under my *right* arm. Sure enough, my right arm was bandaged, not my left, the one with the pebble-sized lump. When I was being wheeled into my room, I said to the orderly, "You guys did the wrong arm."

I could see him studying my chart. His eyes clouded over. "Let me get the doctor."

I don't know how long I waited for the doctor. I was in a morphine-induced cloud. When I managed to blink my eyes open and focus, the doc was standing over me.

"We didn't do the wrong arm," he said, continuing the conversation I'd begun with the orderly. "We found another lump under your right arm."

"How big?"

With his thumb and forefinger, the doctor made a circle the size of a quarter.

"Jesus."

"Yeah," he said.

"Is it—?"

"Waiting for the results," he said.

•   •   •   •   •

You think about dying.

Even before you get the news. The thought creeps into your head, takes a seat, and stays there, the elephant in your brain.

Of course, I've been here before. With Derek. Through all the years he fought for his life, the thought that he might die was always in the back of my mind, a constant presence. Now I'm facing it myself. You have to. "Biopsy" is never a word you associate with a good time.

A few years ago I had a heart attack, which got me thinking seriously about the whole dying thing. I survived that but the thought remained etched in my head. One time, I had a really bad headache before a show. I looked at myself in the makeup mirror and I saw a vein on the side of my head that was bright purple and swollen.

"You see that vein?" I said to a comic who was sitting next to me. "That's really bad. I hope I'm not having a stroke or something. If I am, I hope I can hang on so it doesn't pop until I get home."

The comic looked at me. "What difference does it make where you are? Here, home, on the plane . . . you'll be dead. Why do you care?"

He had a point. But that made me wonder. What would be the best way to die? I asked my doctor.

"Either heart attack or stroke," he said. "No question. Because if you have a big enough stroke, you'll be dead before you hit the floor. That's ideal. You don't want cancer because then you can hang on for years, suffering and everything."

I was still confused. "But if you go suddenly, what happens to your stuff? If I'm at the airport and I have an aneurysm and I fall down dead, what about my bags? I didn't get to claim my luggage. I always have personal things in my bags."

"That's the beauty part. It's not your stuff anymore. You're *dead.* Not your problem."

"This is not working for me. I want to die at home."

"Fine. Just go for a really big stroke or massive heart attack. That way you're out. No pain, no suffering, bang, boom, we're sitting at your funeral."

"Great. Thanks for the tip."

"My pleasure."

His *pleasure?* Where do I find these people?

• • • • •

Back at Mayo. Lying in my hospital bed. My right arm begins to throb. Instinctively, I rotate my shoulder, which sends a painful ping down the entire side of my body. I muffle a howl, remind myself not to do that again. I start to say something to my parents. The door handle clicks, and two doctors step into the room, the doctor who found the lumps and another guy I don't recognize. Their faces are gray from five o'clock shadow and delivering bad news. I see no relief in sight, no light in their eyes.

"Robert," the lump doctor says. I sit up. With a slight flourish, he gestures to the other doctor as if he's the grand prize on a game show. "This is Dr. Mehldau. He's going to be your oncologist."

"Oncologist?" I hear myself say. "You mean I have cancer?"

"Yes," Dr. Mehldau says.

And then, as if I'm in a fever dream, I am far away and I am instantly, monstrously big, and Dr. Mehldau is minute, a speck in a teeny white lab coat. I tower over him, a fifty-foot man, and then, just as quickly, our sizes reverse, and he is fifty feet tall and towering over me. I am delirious, hallucinating, undergoing a mad moment of disconnection. This is not happening to me. This is happening to someone else. I've got too much at stake, too much on the table. These guys have wandered into the wrong room, or misread the chart. I want to scream, *You got the wrong guy!* but nothing feels real. Time has stopped dead and I am both out of my body and out of my mind.

A sound—my mom whimpering? my dad clearing his throat?—shocks me back to the present tense. I know I haven't taken leave of myself for long, but something tells me that the calm in my hospital room is a front, hiding underlying chaos. I have to find my way back to reality and comfort my parents, my protectors. Even though I'm the one with the big *C* stamped on my forehead, I feel I have to protect them. I don't know if they can deal with this.

They've been through so much. First Derek, their grandson, and now me, their son? How are they going to get through this?

Dr. Mehldau steps forward, a foot away from my bed. The other doc allows his hand to rest on my mother's shoulder.

She reaches up and clutches two of his fingers, her other hand entwined with my father's on her lap.

From his lab coat pocket, Dr. Mehldau produces a small yellow legal pad and a Sharpie. He screeches a black line down the middle of the top page. I smell the alcoholic scent of the felt-tipped marker.

"There's Hodgkin's disease." Dr. Mehldau writes and speaks simultaneously, scratching the words *Hodgkin's lymphoma* on one side of the page in clumsy cursive script. "And non-Hodgkin's lymphoma." He scribbles these words on the other side of the black line and looks up at me. "You have non-Hodgkin's lymphoma."

"Just my luck," I say. "I get the one not named after the guy."

Dr. Mehldau laughs, jarringly, then says, "Well, if you can find something funny the moment you get the diagnosis, you're going to be okay."

Poof. The joke brings a moment of relief. Of hope. The tension in the room escapes. It's as if we're encased inside a giant balloon, and, pop, I've stuck a pin in it and let the air out. All that's left now are the five of us and Mr. C, the rampaging rhinoceros in the room.

Amazing when you hear that word.

Cancer.

Cancer.

I know that for some people just hearing "You've got cancer" means they're dead. Bam. Might as well stop at the mortuary on the way home and pick out the casket. Life over. And the buzzer sounds. Ball game.

And I know that there are other people, loved ones, sitting bedside, who immediately say, "Don't worry, you're not going through this alone."

Yeah? When they lower me into the ground, are you jumping in, too? I don't think so. I'm taking this death cruise all by myself. I know that much.

What's strange, but not surprising, is that when I hear the word, my first reaction, my initial instinct, is to go for the laugh.

It really is. I don't plan it, don't think about it. I just go for it. I realize instinctively that even though I've just been told I have cancer, I haven't been told that I'm going to die. And to prove it, I'm going to do the one and only thing that shows that I am very much alive:

I am going to make the audience laugh.

It's a small house tonight—my mom, my dad, the lump doctor, and my oncologist—but they've paid for their tickets (well, it's co-pay). They're here for the show and I'm not going to let them down. I've still got my sense of humor, my edge. And that means I'm alive!

What's even better is that I'm a big hit. Dr. Mehldau, my oncologist, loves it. He gets the joke. Even better, I have the feeling that he gets *me.*

"Yes. If you can keep your sense of humor, you're going to be okay," he says again.

I'm thrilled he says this because my first reaction to the news—going for the laugh—lasts about as long as it takes me to get the joke out. My second reaction kicks in right away, pretty much canceling out the first one.

My second reaction is total shock.

As I said, the thought of dying has crossed my mind. Now here's Dr. Mehldau hitting me with the *C* word, and I remember my doctor in L.A. telling me that I should try to die from a stroke or a heart attack in the middle of the night and not from something like cancer because of all the pain and suffering, and now I'VE GOT CANCER. Guess I screwed that up. And Dr. Mehldau is talking in his low, serious doctor's voice, a kind of gravelly baritone that somehow reminds me of the ninety-year-old cantor who smelled like a musty attic, at the synagogue in New York where I had my bar mitzvah. I'm trying to focus on the words dancing out of Dr. Mehldau's mouth, I'm *trying,* but I'm only picking up every third word: stage one, V cell, large V cell, stage two, D cell, T cell, wait, I remember reading that Mr. T had T-cell lymphoma, which sounded funny at the time and somehow I blink and connect to Dr. Mehldau through my haze and hear him say, "Indolent, which is slow-growing, we can sometimes just watch it, but your cancer is, unfortunately, aggressive—"

Aggressive is not a word I want to hear in the same sentence as *cancer.* Aggressive is a good word for a woman. As in, I've always wanted to be stuck in an elevator with a beautiful, *aggressive* woman with a huge rack and no gag reflex.

Then I go from shock to panic.

I ask Dr. Mehldau, "Aggressive? How aggressive? Am I gonna make it to the parking lot?"

"I'm going to be blunt." Dr. Mehldau holds for a beat. Strangely enough I'm thinking that this can't be that easy for *him*.

"Okay," I say.

"If you went untreated, if we didn't catch this now, now as in *today*, you would be dead in six months."

"But you caught it," I say.

"We caught it," Dr. Mehldau says. "I'm going to put you on chemotherapy starting in two days. That means Wednesday. That gives you exactly one day to get yourself together. Sorry, but that's the way it has to be. By the way, Robert, are you open-minded?"

"I guess you haven't seen my act. Why?"

"Well, some patients find that using marijuana during chemotherapy helps with the nausea and appetite loss. It's actually safer and a lot more mild than most of the anti-nausea injections they give you. So that's an option."

I look over at my mom and dad. No reaction. Just nodding. A reflex. Taking it all in. Trying to *deal*. I look at Dr. Mehldau. He smiles, and I'm thinking—

Did he just say in front of my parents that I could smoke pot? This is a dream come true. Where was he when I was eighteen years old?

And then, whap, I'm back to reality, back to thinking about the chemotherapy, and what could happen.

"Dr. Mehldau, I'm a very positive person, but what if the treatment doesn't work?"

"Honestly? You have six to eight months. If it does work, you have a 51 percent chance of going two years without a reoccurrence. You make it two years, then chances improve greatly that you can make it to five years, which is what we base the survival rate on."

"This is really fucked," I say.

"Well, yeah. But the good news is—"

"I know. See that nurse out there? You're banging her."

Dr. Mehldau laughs, shakes his head. I wink at my parents.

"Old joke," I say. "But if you haven't heard it, it's new."

"The good news is," Dr. Mehldau repeats, "I'm being conservative. I have to be. But if you're stage three, which I'm convinced you are, with the treatment here and your attitude, well, I just have a good feeling."

I swallow, look over at my parents. My mother is wiping her eyes with a tissue. My father is nodding as if he's *davening.*

"What we're gonna do now is a bone marrow biopsy to rule out stage four. Either way, count on starting treatment Wednesday."

"Is there a stage five?" my dad asks.

"Yeah," I say. "A studio development deal."

"So Wednesday," Dr. Mehldau says and pats the blanket next to my leg. "Okay?"

I nod, peek at my parents again. I feel dazed, a fighter who's been sucker-punched and who's just crawled back to his corner. But somehow, like Rocky, the fighter knows that this is *it,* the fight of his life, and I feel an energy shift—call it my survival instinct or my will—and I say to Dr. Mehldau, "You said I have six to eight months if the treatment doesn't work and 51 percent of going two years without it coming back, right?"

"Yes."

"I don't like those two options."

"I know, but—"

"No." I say this too loudly so I lower my voice and say just above a whisper, "There's another option. A third option. And that is that it never comes back."

Dr. Mehldau shifts his weight, and in a whisper echoing mine says, "There is a possibility of that, yes."

"Then that's my choice," I say. "I'm going with number three."

I lock my eyes into his. And instead of lowering his eyes or turning away, he fastens his stare on mine. He is not playing a game and he's not patronizing me. We're in this together. That I know, suddenly and profoundly.

"Then number three it is," he says.

MONDAY AFTERNOON

I'm not ready to die. Period.

To begin with, I cannot imagine a future without me in it. Can't do it. There is no such place. Sorry. I'm still here, in every picture. I look like shit, but I'm here. And I'm gonna keep making people laugh even if I have to stand at the microphone with a quill of IVs poking out of me. I don't care. I'm not going down without a laugh.

I feel like I'm on speed. My life is whirring by. Every second is accelerated. I'm breathless. Gotta slow down. Can't. I feel like I'm riding on a bullet train, my face pressed against the window, the world outside racing past, a blur. Cancer, it seems, fucks you up *fast.*

They talk about the five stages of cancer, same as the five stages of grief. Well, it's really six. Because the first one is shock. The other five are denial, anger, bargaining, depression, and acceptance. Trust me. Each stage is a bitch. What's an even bigger bitch is that they're not necessarily in order and they can overlap. Now, I do have a leg up because being in show business, I've already been through all five stages pretty much on a daily basis. Except for anger. Even when I was at my lowest point, I never went there. I just felt that being pissed off would only muddy my already muddy waters. In other words, what good would it do?

Still in the hospital on D-Day (Diagnosis Day) I have not one but *two* visits from clergymen. The first one is a rabbi. Surprisingly young, thin, pasty-skinned, his too-big yarmulke swimming on him. Looks like he's trying to balance a plate on his head. Very sympathetic eyes.

"How are you?" he says.

"Been better."

He shrugs. Rabbis shrug all the time. Must be part of their yeshiva training. "I can imagine. Well, I *can't* imagine, but I can try." Shrug, shrug.

"The hardest part is accepting that they're talking about *me*," I say. "I keep thinking they're talking about some other guy. I can't have cancer."

"That's human nature," the rabbi says shrugging once, twice. Looks like he's doing some weird penguin dance. He raises a bony finger toward the ceiling. "Your vacuum cleaner breaks, you accept it. A lightbulb burns out, you toss it away, get another one. But when it's us? When we face the Angel of Death? Difficult to accept. Also, we know instinctively that when a lightbulb burns out, the electricity doesn't die."

I smile gravely as if he's just handed me the secret of life. Actually, I don't know what the hell's he's talking about. Lightbulbs? Vacuum cleaners? Does this guy run an appliance store on the side? And if he's so smart, why can't he find a yarmulke that fits?

"Thank you, Rabbi," I say.

"Anytime." He pats my hand like I'm his *bubbie*. "Do you pray?"

"Sometimes. Usually when I want something really bad." I want to say like a Porsche or a blow job but I hold back. Instead I ask him, "Why? Do you think praying really helps?"

"I don't know. But what's the downside?" The rabbi grins, shrugs like a maniac, and leaves.

About an hour later, a chaplain shows up. This guy's decked out in an Armani suit, a string tie, cowboy boots, and has really good hair, black, wavy, and lacquered like he's up for a remake of *Dallas*.

"Mind if I drop in for a visit?"

"Not at all. Come on in."

He flashes a smile as wide as a keyboard. "How are you?"

"Well, you know."

He nods. He plows his fingers through his hairdo. His hair barely moves. Incredible. Maybe the thing is a hair hat. "Do you go to church?"

"Actually I'm Jewish, so, no, not that much."

"Sorry. I hope I didn't offend you by coming in here."

"Are you kidding? I'm not offended at all. I've got cancer. This is not the time for me to play favorites. If Jesus is the main guy, then I'm on his side. I've even dabbled with Buddhism. Because at this point, I'm betting win, place, and show."

The chaplain laughs.

"I'm serious," I say. "I do not want to get up there and have Jesus say, 'I'm gonna sit you down right now and show you how many times people asked you to accept me as your savior and you blew them off. Not so fast with the answers now, are you? You sit over there until the Rapture's done and then we'll get back to you.' Uh-uh. You get the word that you have cancer, you want to cover your bases."

"I hear you. Well, listen, if there's anything you need. Anything you want to discuss. We can talk, I have literature—"

That's when I notice the small rectangular bulge in his shirt pocket. Nice. The chaplain's a Marlboro man.

"There is something you can do for me."

"Certainly. What is it?"

"Can I bum a cigarette off you?"

The chaplain lowers his chin to his chest and eyes the pack of smokes in his pocket. He raises his eyebrows, as if asking himself, "Hey, how did a pack of cigarettes get into my pocket?" then smiles at me conspiratorially.

"Okay. Sure." He whips the Marlboros out of his pocket and taps out a cigarette. I snap it away by the filter.

"Thanks, man."

Chappy smiles, a manly smile, a cowpoke smile. He'd tip his hat if he had one. Then he aims his finger at me. "We'll talk."

I'm tempted to say, "Praise, Jesus," but he's gone. I study the cigarette in my hand. Cancer stick. That's what they call these things. I don't care. I'm dying for a cigarette.

Here's the stupid part.

I don't smoke.

I can't explain it. Maybe I want to tempt Fate. Maybe I want to laugh in cancer's face. I have no idea. I palm the cigarette, pop it into my shirt pocket for later. Maybe I'll smoke it while I polish off a fifth of gin.

Yeah. You got it. I don't drink, either.

* * * * *

The nurse means well.

"We'll see you Wednesday in the infusion center for your first chemo session," she says "Right now, I'm sure you want to go home."

Sounds innocent enough.

I'm sure you want to go home.

I do. I do want to go home.

I'm just not exactly sure where *home* is.

Is home where your heart is?

Or where your family is?

To explain: I'm in love with and am currently living with Melissa. I also love my kids and my parents, still care for Vicki, and I'm currently living with cancer.

What am I going to do?

And then a miracle happens. Or at least something I never expected.

Vicki, who is legally my wife but, as we both know, was about to become my ex-wife, makes an offer that qualifies her for sainthood.

She offers to take care of me. She invites me to her home in Arizona where I can be close to Mayo, my parents, and our children. She volunteers to be my nurse and my caregiver. A remarkable offer. An incredible act of kindness.

"Robert, I know where your heart is," she says. "I know it's in L.A. But this isn't about that. It's about saving your life."

I start to protest. She gently cuts me off.

"We've been through this before, with Derek," she says. "I know what to do. I'm willing to do it again. No strings attached. When you're well, you can move on. I mean it. Think about it."

I do think about it. I agonize over it.

The truth is, everything Vicki's said is right. She nursed Derek and she knows cancer. She knows the questions to ask the doctors, what medications I'll need, the doses, the times, the combinations. She was amazing with Derek. He was diagnosed when he was three years old. The doctors gave him six months to live. He lived for eight years. It was largely due to his indomitable spirit and Vicki's inexhaustible care. As a caregiver, she's the best there is. Nobody touches her.

I also want to be close to our kids. I want to spend as much time as possible with Jessica, Aliyah, and Jacob. In another extraordinary act of kindness, Jessica has said that she will leave college for a semester so she can help take care of me.

I want to be near her and Aliyah and Jacob so I can see them whenever I can. I want to know them and I want them to know me, even if we have only a few more months together.

And I want to be near my parents. They are survivors in the truest sense. They will fight with me, next to me, support me in any and every way they can. I know there is a long, rough road ahead and I will need constant care and supervision.

I don't want to sound patronizing or diminishing, but I just can't lay all of this on Melissa. As much as I love her and as much as I love *us,* I can't do that to her. I can't put her through that. It's not fair to her. This is not what she signed up for. She's twenty-six years old. She really does have her whole life ahead of her. As opposed to me. I may have six months ahead of me. Do I seriously want to die in her apartment in West Hollywood, her burden? As much as it's killing me, I have to end it with her. For her own good. And I'd be lying if I said I wasn't thinking of my own good, too.

I make my decision. I will accept Vicki's offer. I'll double-check first to make sure I wasn't hallucinating and then I'll take her up on it. It is an amazing offer. And it feels like my only choice.

So tomorrow I will fly to L.A. and end it with Melissa. I will break up with the love of my life.

No wonder I need a smoke.

MONDAY NIGHT

I stand outside Vicki's house, in the backyard, soaking up the panoramic view of the mountains and desert. Nice house, too. Roomy, comfortable, well furnished.

Something's wrong with this picture.

The divorce settlement (Divorce number one, was it? Who remembers?) bought her a beautiful home in a desert paradise.

My lawyer managed to scrape up enough of the leftover crumbs so I could afford to rent a one-bedroom rat hole on the fringe of Hollywood. Let's clear up something right now. Cancer is a shafting, but, it's a cakewalk compared to divorce.

As the sun starts to dip behind the last mountain peak, the desert sky turns bright orange, and shafts of maroon and silver light stab the desert floor as if through a giant kaleidoscope. The effect is dazzling, hallucinogenic, nature's nightly light show.

As I watch the sun park itself for the night, I wonder how many more Arizona sunsets I'll see, and I light up the Marlboro. I take a long, deep drag. Within half a second, I choke on the smoke and start coughing nonstop. My throat is on *fire*. I can barely catch my breath, I'm coughing so much.

Finally, I exhale slowly, somehow stifle the coughing, and compose myself. I flip the cigarette over and stare at the burning end. I shake my head. What the hell am I doing? I'm a moron. I'm insane. I have to cut this shit out.

I take another drag.

My throat is *ablaze*. It feels like I've jammed a white-hot poker into my neck. Suddenly, a wave of nausea rises up into the back of my mouth. I take one step and my knees wobble. Man, am I dizzy. The desert is spinning. Lights. Dazzling. Dizzy. The sky is *whirling* around me.

What am I doing? The lymphoma's not enough? I have to start inhaling smoke, too? Is this some sort of reverse psychology or distraction technique? Take my mind off the cancer by smoking a cigarette? Yeah. Great. Makes a lot of sense. That's one thing about cancer. You don't think straight.

Cancer. I have cancer. People die from cancer. My son Derek died from cancer. My grandmother died from it. You know what? *All* of my relatives have died from cancer. This is no bullshit.

I'm dead. I'm really dead. And when you're dead, you're fucking *dead*. Like really *really* dead. Not like in all those dopey movies where people actually see dead people. Forget that. Like at the end of *Ghost* when Patrick Swayze says to Demi Moore, "I love you," and she says, "Ditto."

I wouldn't go, *Ditto*. I'd go, *I thought you were dead! Why am I seeing you? If you're dead, and I'm seeing you, that means I'm dead, too! Holy shit!*

My thoughts are racing. My nose starts to tingle and I'm sweating, dripping sweat, the sweat is leaking out of me, and as the desert turns dark, I feel a shadow creeping toward me, and my hands begin to tremble, and I'm cold, freezing again, and here they come, the shakes, and I realize that suddenly I'm scared, scared shitless, scared that I'm going to die without spending enough time with my kids, and that I will never have the life I've dreamed about with Melissa, and I just feel fucked, and I find myself inside dialing Dr. Mehldau's private number, the phone soaked with my sweat. He answers on the third ring.

"It's Robert. I'm sorry to bother you at home—"

"Robert, what's the matter?"

"What's the matter? I have cancer. I'm really anxious. Really scared. I'm sweating and I'm shaking. I'm freaking out. I need a Valium or a Xanax."

"Absolutely not."

This I don't expect. I shift the phone to my other ear. Clear my throat. "Um. What?"

"No," Dr. Mehldau says.

"Maybe I'm not making myself clear. I'm teetering here. I'm really feeling fucked up and really, *really* scared."

Dr. Mehldau pauses for a millisecond. He speaks slowly, with infinite patience and calm. "I hear you. I do."

"I don't want a whole bottle. I just want one. To get me through the night." I close my eyes, willing the world to stop spinning.

"Why do you want a Valium?" he asks.

"I told you. I'm having an anxiety attack."

"Robert, considering what I told you this afternoon, it's normal to have an anxiety attack. If you weren't feeling incredibly anxious and scared, I'd be worried about you."

"You would?"

"Yeah. I'd think there was something wrong with you. I'd think you didn't care. I'd be concerned that you heard what I said and that you thought of it as a death sentence. I'd be worried that you'd given up."

"So the fact that I'm freaking out is a good thing?"

"Well, kind of, yeah."

"Uh-huh." Now I pause. "I'm talking about one pill—"

"Look, if you were gonna fight Mike Tyson for the heavyweight championship of the world, what would you do?"

"Try to make it to the bathroom without having an accident in public."

"Seriously, what would you do?"

I rub my left eye, which is now throbbing. "I don't know."

Mehldau pushes on. "You'd hire a trainer and a corner man, wouldn't you? And a nutritionist, and a sparring partner, and you'd do road work every day, and you'd get videotapes of him fighting and you'd study him. You'd do everything you could to prepare so that when you stepped into the ring for the fight of your life, you'd know all his strengths and weaknesses. Would you do all that?" He holds for a beat. "Or would you take a Valium?"

"No," I say. "I would do all that."

"Well, hang up with me, and go on the Internet and start reading all about non-Hodgkin's lymphoma. And when you're at Mayo, go to the library and do research. Find ways to help you get through it. Read other people's stories. Find out how you're gonna beat it. Become an expert."

I murmur, "Knowledge is power, right?"

"Exactly," Dr. Mehldau says.

I feel my breathing slow down. My hands have stopped trembling and my body temperature has returned to normal. I no longer feel as if I'm trapped inside an ice chest. A sense of calm washes over me. I know what I have to do. Dr. Mehldau has not only relaxed me, he has given me a game plan.

Since my cancer is aggressive, I have to be aggressive, too. In order to fight, I have to know *what* I'm fighting. I have never been a passive person and I'm not going to start now. I refuse to lay back and let the cancer take over. I'm going after it. That will be my new purpose.

Talk about life throwing you a curve ball. Yesterday I fantasized that in six months I'd be known as Robert Schimmel, sitcom star. Today I'm fantasizing that in six months I'll be alive. Amazing how fantasies change. Wasn't long ago that my fantasies involved me and two women in cheerleader outfits.

"Robert?" Dr. Mehldau says.

"Huh?"

"You there?"

"Yeah. I was just thinking about what you were saying. I'm taking it in. The news today? Blindsided me a little bit."

"I know. Look, I can give you a Valium tonight, but tomorrow morning when you wake up, you're still gonna have cancer and you won't have any Valium. And instead of dealing with your disease, you're avoiding it. You have cancer, Robert. You have to embrace it. That's how you deal with it. Sounds weird, but it's true."

I don't say anything. I hold the phone close, cradle the receiver.

"You okay, Robert?"

"Yeah. Considering."

"I know. Listen, I'm here. You can call me anytime. I mean that."

"Thank you. Hey, Dr. Mehldau?"

"Yes?"

"Will you be my corner man?"

I can feel his smile through the phone.

TUESDAY

9:35 a.m. Leaving Arizona, heading to L.A. aboard Southwest Airlines. The desert below is the color of rust. My mission in L.A. consists of two brutal tasks.

One: inform my manager that I have cancer and that I have to walk away from my own television show, the career opportunity of a lifetime. No problem. Only waited twenty-five years for this. My manager has stuck with me through the worst bullshit you can imagine. Guy's a saint. This news should send him screaming right into the street.

Two: tell Melissa that I'm breaking up with her and that I'm never going to see her again.

The only good thing about Number Two is that it makes Number One seem like a piece of cake.

The flight from Phoenix to L.A. takes a little more than an hour, but it feels like a day and a half. The landing is rocky. I barely notice. Funny how things that used to make me crazy suddenly don't even make a dent. Like turbulence on a plane. So the plane bounces a little because one of the flight attendants is blowing the pilot. Who cares? I stayed up until three in the morning poring over information about non-Hodgkin's lymphoma on the Web. Tons of stuff to learn. Of course, I was fascinated by those who didn't make it.

Jackie Kennedy Onassis, for one, died from non-Hodgkin's lymphoma. Doesn't matter how rich or famous you are, cancer is an equal opportunity shit sandwich.

First stop, my manager Lee's office. The receptionist smiles, asks, "How's it going, Robert?" I resist the urge to launch into the events of the past twenty-four hours. Nothing gained by making other people uncomfortable, so I mutter, "Fine, great," and try to smile. Thankfully, Lee appears right away and steers me down the hall into his office. He closes the door. I've already given him the headlines on the phone. I fill him in on the details. He listens quietly, making a tent with his fingers. We've been through a lot of crap together, but this latest pile towers over everything else.

"Obviously, I can't do the show, Lee. I know how hard you've worked for this. I'm really sorry."

He blinks with a mixture of surprise and sadness. "Robert, the show doesn't matter. This is about your health. It's about getting well. I don't care about the show."

I know this is show business, the loneliest and most vicious business in the world, but Lee's reaction touches me. He is a genuinely kind and supportive person. A *mensch*.

"What happens now?" I ask him.

He shrugs. "A holding pattern. The network will have to put on something else. I mean, the show is called *Schimmel.* It's all about *you.* They can't retool it."

"What if they try to replace me with somebody else?"

"Like who? There's nobody else like you."

"I don't know. You know how they think. They'll go with Erik Estrada."

Lee smiles, shakes his head, then blows out a sigh that could pass as a moan. "What a difference a day makes. Yesterday, June 4th, you had the world by the balls. HBO special, CD deal, sitcom on the air. The hat trick. Twenty-fours later, June 5th, the bomb drops. Boom."

"Yeah. The Schimmel Touch," I say. "The Midas Touch in reverse. Everything I touch turns to shit."

Lee stands up, shakes his head, not disagreeing. He allows a small, ironic smile.

"I'm sorry, Lee," I say again. "I know this is a kick in the nuts."

"Robert, your job now is to get better, period," Lee says. "We'll have other chances. You're a fighter. It's gonna be all right."

We hug. A long, silent embrace. More than manager and client who are fond of each other. More than two close friends who've shared the same foxhole and fought the show business wars shoulder to shoulder. More like two brothers.

And then, as we cling to each other, Lee murmurs in a soft, low voice, "Just take care of yourself, Robert."

●　●　●　●　●

Now for the hard part.

Breaking up with Melissa.

I've figured out what I'm going to say. Practiced it. Got it down.

I'm gonna tell her I'm gay.

Ah, she'll never buy it. Plus I think she'll want to try to cure me.

I need to slow down. Think this through. And with my life currently whizzing by me at the speed of light, I desperately need to keep everything from careening out of control and crashing. But for some reason this conversation is one I can't plan. Every time I try to write my "goodbye, Melissa" speech in my mind, my brain locks. Refuses to allow the words to form. Won't let me go there.

I believe in signs. Symbols. Should've seen the signs at all three of my weddings with Vicki. The signs weren't exactly subtle. I'm talking about huge neon yellow caution signs flashing right in my eyes, blinding me. Somehow I didn't notice them.

Wedding number one. A justice of the peace presides, a nervous woman in a powder blue suit. She speed-reads our vows through thick half-glasses, her face tight, her lips barely moving. She finishes, breaking some kind of land speed record for completing the marriage vows.

"Congratulations," she says, packing up her purse. "You can kiss each other, whatever."

"Would you mind signing the marriage license?" I ask her.

"Can't," she says. "I'm late. I was supposed to be in the courtroom down the hall. I'm getting a divorce. I hope you guys have better luck than I did."

I'd call that a sign. Missed it. A few months later we had that one annulled.

Wedding number two. Las Vegas. We go for *kitsch*. We hit a wedding chapel and are hitched by an Elvis impersonator. Lot of "Love Me Tender" references flying around, but I should've known that this was a sign that we'd be impersonating a marriage. Couple years later, "Heartbreak Hotel." Divorce.

Wedding number three is the biggie. A sign here about as obvious as the burning bush, only, again, I don't see it.

This time we're married by a rabbi. The ceremony is trucking along smoothly, no glitches. Everything's cool until the rabbi, a world-class shrugger, tells me to break the glass, which is the final leg of the wedding ceremony, right before we kiss to seal the deal. I stomp on the hidden shot glass, a tiny mound swathed in a cloth napkin. Only the glass won't break. I slam my foot down a second time. The glass feels like a lump of concrete under the heel of my leather shoe. Now I lift my knee as high as I can to crush the thing a third time as if I'm making wine. Nothing. By now, the wedding guests are laughing.

"What happens if I can't break the glass?" I ask the rabbi.

He shrugs in concern. "You *must* break the glass. According to tradition, smashing the glass symbolizes destroying any bad luck that's surrounding your marriage. You want to get rid of the Evil Eyes, don't you?"

I whisper, "You say Evil Eyes. I call them my in-laws." Big-time rabbinical shrug, stifling a laugh this time. After a jab in my side from Vicki's elbow, I say loud enough to get a laugh, "Rabbi, you wouldn't happen to have some dynamite, would you?"

I manage to crunch the glass on my fourth try. Everybody applauds, mostly from relief.

Cut to today: my marriage wrecked, my body wracked with cancer. Should've realized that not being able to break that glass was a giant biblical sign.

•   •   •   •   •

It's early Tuesday afternoon by the time I get to my apartment. I'm feeling drained and dizzy. I wander through my apartment, a zombie, tossing the few remnants of my life in L.A. into my suitcase: some books and CDs, a couple of shirts, sweatpants, and framed photographs of my kids. One picture is of Derek and me. He's sitting in my lap. I'm smiling and he's laughing, no doubt at something silly I've said. He was always my best audience. I really believe his sense of humor helped him through his cancer treatments. It's stunning when I think about it. Derek was happy most of the time. Even through the worst of it, the most debilitating and painful procedures, he managed to keep upbeat. I learned so much from him. So much. I caress his face in the photograph.

And then I dial the phone.

Melissa picks up on the second ring. I barely wait for her to answer. I speak breathlessly. I let out my words as gently as I can, but I know what I'm saying is striking her, hitting her like a bomb. For me, it's yet another explosion in twenty-four hours of nonstop explosions. I hear myself acting, trying to make her believe such half-truths as "I'm too old for you," "I'm not being fair to you," "I want to try again with Vicki for the sake of the kids," and the most bullshitty of all bullshit reasons, "I need space."

After I spew out my long goodbye, Melissa says nothing for what seems like an hour. Then she says, "This doesn't even sound like you, Robert. I'm coming over."

Before I can argue or stop her, she clicks off. I stand stranded in my bare-bones living room, a stranger in my own skin, feeling beyond horrible, feeling suddenly sick, spent, exhausted. Within seconds it seems, my intercom buzzer echoes through the empty apartment.

"Robert, let me in."

"Melissa, please understand," I say through the intercom. "I have to end it. I have to."

"Why? I don't get it. You're not telling me everything."

"No, I am. I really am. I have to move on with my life and you have to, too. Let's just leave it at that. Please."

Everything I say sounds so hollow, so full of crap. No way Melissa's buying any of it. I feel like such a heel.

"What did I do?" She's desperately trying to figure this out, trying to make some sense of it. "Did I do something to you?"

"No, no, you didn't do anything."

"Robert—"

She's crying now, sobbing. I can't leave her like that in the lobby. I buzz her up. Time now shimmers and all I know is that she's upstairs with me and I'm holding her, smelling her hair, and her tears are streaming down her cheeks onto my shirt. I can barely find my voice, but inside I'm silently screaming, *It's not about you. It's not about us. I have cancer. I need to be in Arizona with my kids, my parents, and, yes, Vicki. I need to fight it there and you can't be part of that fight. It's too much for you.*

And I suppose if I were being truly honest, I would have to add, *It's also too much for me.*

And then there is silence as the two of us look at each other, look right into each other's souls. Then we turn away. This, too, this end, is a kind of death.

"What am I supposed to do?" Melissa says. "Just walk out of here and forget about you?"

"You have to," I say and mean it, but then add in a canned, tinny voice: "You deserve somebody better. A younger guy."

She glares at me, her eyes tiny blue dots of rage. "You are so full of *shit*."

I can't say anything because she's right. I am full of shit. I'm also full of heartbreak, loss, guilt, regret, pain, and terror. Plain, simple, unadulterated *fear*. With a capital F. Not the fear of dying, believe it or not, at least not at this moment. The fear that I have made the biggest mistake of my life. And the realization that I can do nothing about it.

"I'm gonna go." Melissa stands straight as a sergeant and then her face creases. She suddenly looks very small and very sad. "Can I at least call you?"

"It'd be better if you didn't."

She nods, her eyes welling up. And then time slows. There is a quick clumsy hug, the door opening but not closing, and the sound of her footsteps clattering down the stairs. I teeter, feeling dizzy again, certain that I will fall. I reach behind me and lean against my rented living room couch for balance. I sit down slowly and exhale massively. I feel a sudden sharp jab in my chest as if I've been knifed, then I gasp for air, caused by the newly formed hole in my heart.

SESSION TWO

"FINDING YOUR PURPOSE"

TUESDAY EVENING

Back in the air.

L.A. to Phoenix.

Winging to my first chemotherapy support group meeting tonight at seven. This should be a hoot.

Okay, just for fun, let's run through my recent little life change one more time.

In twenty-four hours I've gone from a sitcom star on Fox to a cancer patient in Phoenix. I've switched from trying to begin a life with Melissa to trying to save my life at Mayo.

Talk about whiplash. My head's spinning like Linda Blair's in *The Exorcist*.

And I'm feeling—

That's really it, isn't it? That's what being alive is.

Feeling.

Right now I'm feeling numb. In a trance. My head throbbing. As if someone's swatted me across the skull with a tire iron.

But even in this zoned-out zombie state, even as I literally deal with death, I know that my attitude about life has changed.

I feel liberated in a way. But mainly I feel that I have to keep going. I'm going to beat this. I have to. I want to spend time with my kids. I want them to know me. And not just for the next six months. For years to come. I want to watch Jacob and Aliyah grow up and I want them to watch me grow old.

And I'm going to beat this because I want to reconnect with Melissa. Somehow, some way. Maybe we're meant to be. Maybe we're Fated. My head is foggy, but that's not why I think that. At heart, I'm actually a goofy romantic. I cry at Cialis commercials. Especially when the guy thinks he's about to get laid and his grandkids show up. What a bummer. But thank God he's using the dick picker upper that lasts for thirty-six hours. Because if he's using the four-hour one, it's a whole other story. He's got to get those kids out right away or explain why Grandpa's got a baseball bat in his pants.

Thinking about my life now, it boils down to this:

I have to make a comeback. A comeback from cancer.

So where do I start?

Might as well start tonight at the chemotherapy support group.

I don't know what to expect. Don't really expect anything. I just know that the people there are my kind of people— cancer patients—and in my newfound determination to learn everything and anything I can about my disease, I want to go in open-minded.

I am going to face my cancer head-on.

• • • • •

A nondescript room in the back corner of Mayo. People straggle in slowly, heavily, find spots on folding chairs. Nobody bounds in like they've come to hear exercise tips or investment advice. It's a different kind of vibe, an odd combo of hope and despair. A lot of nervous coughing and laughing. I scan the room, trying to get my bearings. I do a head count, which isn't easy because almost everyone is bald. I keep counting the same heads over again. I finally come up with eight, including me. I expect a group leader, but there isn't one. We introduce ourselves and call out our respective cancers. One guy, testicular, tells us that he was diagnosed five years ago and now he's skiing and snowboarding and skydiving. I choke up when he speaks. I vow that that's going to be me. Minus the skiing and snowboarding and skydiving.

Then another guy says in a flat dead voice that he too has non-Hodgkin's lymphoma. He was out three years, everything was cool, and then—

He turns his head and shows us a massive jagged scar, right out of *Planet of the Apes*.

"Yeah," he says. "It came back."

Oh, God, I think. *That's gonna be me.*

I want to get out of here. This was a bad idea. What was I thinking? The panic is starting to stir in my gut—

Somehow I fight it. I beat it down. I can't go there. I can't do the *what ifs* and the *I'm not gonna make its*. I *can't*.

The woman next to me whimpers and starts to cry. The *Planet of the Apes* guy has sucked the life out of the room. He's like a Hoover. I have to change the energy in here. I have to turn it around. I have to do the only thing I know how to do.

Make them laugh. Even once.

"I have non-Hodgkin's lymphoma, too," I say tentatively. "But that's a walk in the park compared to going through a divorce. I can beat cancer." A group giggle. "Cancer goes into remission. Divorce lawyers never stop."

Big laugh. The mood shifts, lightens. We open up. We talk about getting the news, how shocked we felt, how helpless, how we refused to believe it, and then how we gradually accepted the truth because we had no other choice. Cancer is part of us now. We talk about the earliest tests we've gone through. I tell them about my first CAT scan.

"The nurse asked me, 'Are you allergic to squid ink?'"

I hold. They laugh in anticipation.

"How do you know? Seriously. Is it on my birth certificate or do I have to drink squid ink to find out?"

Squeals of laughter now. Testicular Cancer Guy is roaring. I'm hoping he doesn't blow out his good ball.

"They give you iodine in the CAT scan," I say. "Then the nurse says, 'You're gonna feel this sensation. You're gonna taste it, smell it, and then you're gonna feel this warmth go through your body. It usually starts in your head, then travels all through your body. You're really gonna feel it in your crotch.'"

The laughter is rising, going where I hope it will. I hope I'm reading this crowd right.

"Then the nurse says, 'You're gonna have the sensation that you're peeing in your pants. But you're not really peeing in your pants.' And I say, 'What if I really do pee in my pants?'"

A communal roar. I keep going. "'What's that gonna feel like? What kind of sensation is that?' She says, 'No sensation. I guess you'll just find out later.' Great. So it's like a wet dream without the sex?'"

They're gone. Howling. They need this. They need the distraction, the change of pace, the release.

And, honestly, so do I.

WEDNESDAY, JUNE 7, 2000

My first chemotherapy session.

I walk into the infusion center at Mayo, a large, drab room that feels like the inside of a tomb but without the charm. There are a few beds and several chairs arranged near the center, pretty much scrambled together. Behind the cluster of beds and chairs are doors leading off to private rooms where patients with compromised immune systems receive their treatments. The air in here is thick and smells of Lysol. People trudge to their seats as if they are underwater.

The first thing I notice when I walk in is a poster on the back wall of the evolution of man. Except I imagine it in reverse. The *first* image is of a healthy man, walking erect. In each successive frame the man becomes more and more bent over and decrepit. I see myself morph into the poster, becoming over the next eight months the man in the final frame, once strong and healthy, who now looks like a human skeleton.

I scan the room and the images in the poster become suddenly, frighteningly real. *Everyone* in here is the man in the last frame. All the people I see are hooked up to IVs and everybody is either bald or has patches of hair missing. The door to a private room swings open and a man appears in the doorway. He can barely stand. His skin is chalk white. He is bone thin, a walking corpse. He shuffles forward, nods to a nurse, and I think, *I hope to God that was his* last *treatment.*

"Mr. Schimmel?"

A nurse in blue scrubs approaches, extends her hand. She is young, blonde, and cute. More than cute. She's *hot.* Even in her blue crinkly hospital get-up, I can see that she has a *great* body. Man, those feelings never go away. I'm about to have chemotherapy, I'm scared shitless, but a hot blonde calls my name, and I'm thinking maybe I can bang her before the nausea sets in. That's normal, right?

"Please, call me Robert." I give her a smile that could melt the sun, but she spins away and leads me to the beds and chairs where a dozen people are hooked up, getting chemo. Some are lying down, watching TV. A few are sitting up, reading. Some are sleeping. Others are staring off, their eyes vacant.

"You can sit anywhere you like," the nurse says. Her voice is soft and musical. "Or you can lie down—"

"No," I say, surprised at how determined by voice sounds. "I'm not taking this lying down. I'm not giving in to it."

The cute nurse smiles, points to an empty chair.

"Thanks," I say as if she's the hostess leading me to a power table at Spago. "Maybe *thanks* isn't the right word."

She smiles again and starts fiddling with a nearby IV tube. I land in a chair next to a burly guy around my age. His eyes are sunken and his lips are dotted with sores. He looks pissed off.

"I'm Robert."

"Bill." He spits it out. Not sure if he hates his name, me, or life in general.

"How you doing?" I say.

"How do you think I'm doing?" Bill's voice is raspy, his Midwestern drawl a bitter twang. "I got *cancer*."

I look at him. "So do I."

Bill stares back, his sunken eyes lasered into mine. "Good for you."

"Well, I wouldn't call it *good*—"

A brush on my arm. The cute nurse in the blue smock. She speaks low, like a ventriloquist, barely moving her lips. "Maybe you should find another seat. He has a really bad attitude. You need a lot of positive energy to get through this."

I look over at Bill. He glares at me again, then turns away, focusing his attention on a nurse on his left side who's hooking him up to an IV.

"I'm okay," I say. "I like this seat." I smile at Bill. He doesn't smile back. He clears his throat and *clucks,* a dismissive, guttural sound that sends me a clear message: *Don't talk to me. Stay away from me. I want to be left alone.*

That's the message that Bill sends.

It's not the message I receive.

Because in that moment, a lot of things *click.* Immediate things. Life-changing things.

First, even though I've just watched my career land with a splash in a giant toilet, I'm not bitter, and I'm not feeling like I got reamed. I've never been jealous of any other comedian's success. I never say, *Why them? Why not me?* Sometimes it's just the luck of the draw. I know that a lot of comics bitch about other comedians, saying stuff like, *How the hell does he get to film an HBO special at Madison Square Garden while I'm playing Uncle Fucko's Comedy Hutch in Des Moines, Iowa?*

It's timing. In my case, bad timing. The Schimmel Touch. I was on the verge of making it big when I got cancer. I didn't do anything to screw myself up or cause my cancer. And I don't think getting cancer is a punishment or bad karma paying me back for all the bad things I've done in my life. I just don't equate negativity with punishment.

There are people who say, "You cheated on your wife. And see? You got cancer."

I look at them and say, "Really? If you believe in God, do you think that's the way God is? Because if you do, three-quarters of the population would be dead."

Getting cancer is a dose of bad luck. It's walking down the street whistling a happy tune, taking in the fresh air, looking at the clear blue sky, and then stepping in a huge steaming pile of dog shit. That's what cancer is. Getting caught in a drive-by. Your plane going down. Hitting Lotto then getting busted by the I.R.S. for not paying your taxes.

Makes you want to keep your eye on the ball. Makes you want to define your priorities in a hurry. Smell the roses? You bet. Spend time with your kids? Every second I'm with them is precious.

And cancer makes you redefine success. If I based my success on Hollywood standards, I'd say I'm a failure. I'm a snail eating trash at the bottom of the food chain. I don't have a Porsche or a plasma TV or a Rolex.

What do I need? That's the question. Not what do I need to *have,* to *attain,* to *possess.* What do I need to *live?*

Love. True love.

And I need to make people laugh.

That's what fuels me, feeds me, stirs my soul. Making people laugh defines me. Not my bank account or a BMW or a bunch of Tiffany trinkets. Looking around the infusion center, I don't see a parking space for a BMW next to any of the beds. All the money in the world can't buy you health or one more minute of life. And at three in the morning, when you're freaking out, scared shitless that the treatment's not working, who are you going to call to talk you down, your doctor or your BMW dealer?

As the cute nurse with the fabulous body pokes my forearm in search of a willing vein in which to stab the IV, I think, crazily, that I'm actually a lucky man. In every sense of the word. It was unlucky to get cancer. Grant you that. But I am lucky to do what I do for a living. When it's time to do a show, I never say, *Do I really have to go up there and tell these jokes?* I'm thrilled that I get paid to make people laugh.

I look at it that I'm on a temporary hiatus from playing comedy clubs. Taking a little break. This is my club now: The Infusion Room. The toughest room I've ever played. Rough crowd. Made up of people like Bill, not the most receptive guy in the world. Doesn't seem like he's really in the mood to laugh.

That just makes it more of a challenge.

Something tells me that Bill and people like him are the ones who need to laugh the most. I want to try. I want to connect to him. I want to make him smile.

Because when you're laughing, you forget everything else, if just for that five seconds.

Gonna start by warming him up.

"Cancer," I say. "Talk about a shit sandwich, huh?"

Bill turns to me, his face locked in an iron frown. "The nurse is right. You should find another seat."

"This is fine." I wriggle in my chair, trying to find a comfortable position. "So are you going to any support group meetings?"

He grimaces, maybe from the needle that's been plunged into his arm, or maybe from me. "I don't believe in that. It's a waste of time."

"Really?"

"This must be your first treatment, right?"

"Yeah."

"Talk to me after you've had about three treatments and tell me how great the support group meetings are then. They're bullshit."

My mind clamps onto last night's meeting. Pictures of faces flickering by. I remember something. A woman. My instinct goes there, and I say, "I went last night because I wanted to be prepared for what I would face here."

Bill rolls his eyes.

"There was a woman there last night. Kinda ugly. She was crying hysterically and she said, 'I'm gonna have one of my breasts removed and I'm afraid my husband isn't going to find me sexy anymore.' I'm looking at her and I'm thinking, 'Lady, you wouldn't be sexy if you had three tits.'"

Bill's bottom lip quivers, then his mouth cracks open and—he can't help himself—he starts to laugh. The laugh builds to a roaring, out-of-control cackle. Bill's laughing so hard that the cute blonde nurse rushes over to see if he's all right.

"Bill? You okay?" He's doubled over. He waves her away. Then grinning widely, she says to me, "I've never even seen him smile. What did you say to him?"

"I told him about us," I say.

She swats me lightly on the shoulder, then bends over and kisses me on top of the head.

SESSION THREE

"GETTING SICK"

TEN DAYS LATER

You don't get sick right away.

My problem is I've seen a lot of movies where people get cancer and it seems that they're throwing up the second after they start chemo. That's what I expected, anyway. I figured right after the nurse yanked the IV out of my arm, waves of nausea would start hitting me, and I'd be puking in the car on the way home. It's not like that at all.

I get home and I feel fine. No nausea, dizziness, nothing. In fact, I take a brisk thirty-minute walk, which makes me feel refreshed. When I get back, Dr. Mehldau is on the phone.

"Hey, Robert. Thought I'd check in. How you feeling?"

"I feel pretty good. No nausea. This isn't bad at all."

Then one word that's like a stop sign.

"Wait."

"Really?"

"I hate to burst your bubble, but you will get sick. It usually takes between nine and eleven days for your white and red blood cell count to plummet. Then it hits you. That's why we space the chemo treatments three weeks apart. Otherwise you couldn't take it. Nobody could."

"Nice. Thanks. Something to look forward to."

"Sorry." He pauses. "I want to tell you something. Actually, I want you to do something for me."

"All right—"

"I want you to concentrate on *you*. Just you. You're sick. You come first."

"Okay, but when I do, the girl usually gets pissed."

Dr. Mehldau laughs, a short sudden burst, then he stops and pauses for a long beat. "Robert, I really mean it. You need to put yourself first. Do you understand?"

I actually don't. "I have kids," I say.

"That's right, you do. But you're not worth anything to them dead." His words jolt me. I squeeze my eyes shut, listening intently. "Is Vicki a good mom?"

"She's a great mom."

"I knew that. Let her take over completely. You take care of yourself. You have to kick everybody out of your head except you. You've been there for other people before. Now it's time for other people to be there for you. This is important, Robert. Be selfish. You're gonna have to be."

I'm not sure how long I take to respond. It must be a while because Dr. Mehldau speaks first. "Robert?"

"I'm here. I'm thinking about what you said. It's just so weird for me to think that way. It's unnatural."

"Think of it this way," Dr. Mehldau says. "I'm your doctor and I'm giving you a prescription. *Be selfish*."

• • • • •

Dr. Mehldau hits the number on the head. On day ten a coughing jag wakes me at 5 a.m., a hacking, knifing cough that doubles me over, then sends me bolting into the bathroom, arms cradling my stomach before the cough brings me to my knees, bowing and retching into the bowl. Since drinking too much Southern Comfort one Saturday night my junior year of high school, I haven't been a big fan of vomiting. I've heard of bulimic people who eat anything and everything they want because later they'll just make themselves throw up. They can't be Jews.

Lying in a heap on the bathroom floor, waiting for the next wave to hit, I think about my TV show *Schimmel,* the hot new fall sitcom ten days ago, now a videotape gathering dust on some shelf. Before we shot the show, the entire cast had to be examined by a studio doctor for insurance reasons. After my physical, the doctor gave me a totally clean bill of health, compared with the Mayo Clinic, which gave me six months to live. Yeah. The studio guy didn't miss by much. Maybe he wasn't a doctor. Maybe he just played one on TV.

Ohhhh. Here we go again. Excuse me.

*   *   *   *   *

Chemotherapy works the same way as boot camp. I know because I've been through both. Back in the day, when I was eighteen, there used to be a draft lottery. Of course, my luck, the Schimmel Touch, I got number four or something, so I enlisted in the air force. Fortunately, they kicked me out after a year when I ditched K.P. and went AWOL to the movies. True story.

But the philosophy behind both boot camp and chemotherapy is to push you to your limit, kick you to the edge of death, and then back away. It's a simple plan: kill the cancer and try not to kill the patient. Curled up on the tile floor of the can, my head propped against the porcelain base of the toilet bowl, I know that if I survive the chemo, I will beat this fucking cancer. I will.

A few days before I'm scheduled for my second chemo treatment, after the vomiting has run its course, I stand at the kitchen sink, drinking a glass of juice, and I feel something burning in my mouth all the way into my throat. Later I'm in the bathroom taking a crap (well, where else would I take a crap?), and I feel the burning again, only this time it's deeper, burning from my mouth practically all the way down my back. I call Dr. Mehldau, who tells me, with alarm in his voice, to come over to his office right away.

"Wow. You've got a ton of open sores in your mouth," Dr. Mehldau says, peering inside my mouth with a penlight. He snaps off the tiny flashlight. "It's a common side effect." Astride a padded stool with wheels, he rolls himself over to a file cabinet and rummages through one of the drawers. "Throw away your toothbrush. And forget flossing. That's out of the question."

"I can't brush my teeth?"

"Nope. With those sores, if you brush your teeth using a conventional toothbrush, your gums will definitely bleed. If you get an infection while your blood cell count is down, you're dead."

I'm starting to realize that everything this guy says is followed by the words *"You're dead."* As in:

"If you brush your teeth, you're dead."

"If you cut yourself, you're dead."

"If you catch a cold, you're dead."

I sigh, feeling suddenly winded. "You wouldn't think that dental floss could be so hazardous."

"If you floss, you're dead."

"Listen, Dr. Mehldau, you don't know me, but when it comes to hygiene, I'm a little over the top. I have to keep my teeth clean."

"I kind of figured that. Here we go."

He pulls out a handful of small sponges attached to thin wooden sticks. They look like giant fluffy Q-Tips. "Start with these. The nurses at Mayo will keep you supplied. Now. About those sores."

Dr. Mehldau leans forward and fixes me right in the eye. "Robert, you have to avoid all oral and anal contact. That can be very, *very* dangerous. Okay?"

Now, I know I'm pretty outrageous and everything, but at that moment all I can think is: *Do I look like an ass eater to him? Is that how people see me? I do get crazy in my act, but does he think I really do this stuff?*

"Wow," I say aloud. "What a blow. The cancer's not bad enough. Now I can't lick anyone's asshole. When is the punishment gonna stop?"

Dr. Mehldau lifts both eyebrows, and then starts laughing. A fierce cartoon chuckle. Someday I'd love to fill an audience with laughers like that.

"I'm *serious*," he says, but he's laughing.

"I know, I know. If I eat somebody's ass, I'm dead."

"No anal. And no oral."

"No licking, no eating. Got it. What about blow jobs?"

Dr. Mehldau is laughing too much to speak. He manages to shake his head and wag a finger.

"Finally some good news for my wife," I say.

By now Dr. Mehldau's loud scary laugh has dissolved into a kind of frightening silent spasm. I keep going. "So oral sex is out, right?"

"Right."

"Got it," I say. "I don't think either one of us wants to have this conversation again. I'm sure the last thing you want to see is a mouthful of sores again in a week and have to ask me, 'Robert, did you go down on your wife?'"

"Right," he says again. "You can't do that. Not during chemo. You never know what's down there."

I look at him. "You never know what's down there? *I* was down there. Who do you think I'm gonna find down there? Yoda?"

He suddenly stands and waves at me in surrender. He leans briefly against the doorjamb, waves again, and without another word, leaves the room.

Wow. No oral sex. It does make you think. If you shouldn't be doing it now, why should you ever do it? It's like when a woman gets pregnant, the doctor always says, "Don't eat sushi. You shouldn't eat raw fish when you're pregnant because if there's a parasite in it, you're dead." Well, why would you ever eat raw fish?

Same thing with swordfish. Doesn't make sense. If you're not pregnant, you can eat all the swordfish you want. You can fuck the swordfish. But if you're pregnant, forget it. This kind of shit makes me nervous.

That's why when I eat swordfish, I always wear a condom.

•   •   •   •   •

The first chemotherapy session brings me to my knees, knocks me down, but not out. I stagger back to my feet and come back strong, ready for round two. I walk into the infusion center with a box of doughnuts and a chip on my shoulder. *Feeling a teeny bit cocky, Mr. Chemo. I can handle you. You rocked me, but you couldn't close the deal.* Seven sessions to go. I know I can go the distance.

The nurses are all over the doughnuts. Makes me happy. I'm thrilled to be the one to provide them with their mid-morning sugar high. They're really the unsung heroes in all this, caring for people whose bodies, minds, and emotions are being devastated on a daily basis. It takes a special type of person to work with cancer patients. I'm taking what Dr. Mehldau said to heart—I am going to try to be a little selfish—but I know I'll feel better about myself if I can make their jobs a little easier by (a) not being the asshole patient (there's one in every infusion center; if you don't know who it is, it's you), and (b) getting them to laugh.

As I wander through the heart of the room, I spot Bill, formerly the asshole patient, who's waving frantically at me and pointing to a chair he's saved next to him. I weave over to him and plant myself on the seat.

He smiles. "How you doing?"

"How do you think I'm doing? I got cancer."

Bill chuckles. The cute blonde nurse, whose name I've learned is Nadine, arrives and hooks me up to my IV. While she's poking around for an available vein, Bill smiles at her, too. She's so shocked she nearly jabs the IV into her own arm.

"Nice kid," Bill says after she's done. "Okay, you ready?"

"For what?"

"To laugh. I got jokes, man."

And Bill begins peppering me with dozens of puns, jokes, and one-liners he's collected, his face reconfigured from his previously permanent scowl to a disarming smile and a constant twinkling of his eyes. At one point, before Bill's big finish, Nadine walks by holding a jelly doughnut, her fingers dusted with powdered sugar.

"How's your day going, Nadino?" he says. Big smile.

"Fine," she says. "How about you, Bill? How's your day going?"

"I've had worse. Probably gonna have worse, too. Hey, I got a joke for you."

"Bring it on."

She fastens me with a huge, thankful smile. After the punch line, she laughs and leaves and Bill polishes off his routine. Suddenly we get serious and talk about the side effects he's suffered. His choice of topic.

"I want you to be prepared for what's down the road," Bill says solemnly, but without bitterness. I thank him and tell him about Dr. Mehldau warning me about the hazards of oral sex. I mention the dangers associated with eating somebody's ass.

"He never warned me about that," Bill says. "But then again, you look like an ass eater."

"You know, you're getting a little too funny," I say. "Maybe you should go back to being a dick."

"Too late, Robert. You cured me," Bill says, by far the nicest thing anyone's said to me all day. Hell, almost any day.

• • • • •

Two nights later, my hair falls out at dinner. Just like that. No warning. Bam. Like a nuclear shower hitting a fir tree full blast and knocking every needle off, zap, leaving nothing but naked branches.

I'm poking at my food, sitting across the table from Vicki, contemplating yet again the whiplash known as my life, and while contemplating, I absently begin rubbing my chin, which, until that moment, had been covered with a neatly trimmed and manicured goatee. My fingers feel moist and scratchy. I look down and my food is completely covered in chin hair.

"Holy shit." I'm more amazed than angry. I stare at my plate. "Wow. What's for dinner, honey? How about a big bowl of *hair*?"

Since starting chemo, I'd been expecting to lose my hair. I just never expected it to all fall out at once, like a massive brown snowfall. I head into the bathroom to check out my face in the mirror. Sure enough, most of the hair on my chin is gone. Basically what's left is my mustache.

I turn on the faucet, cup my hands under the water, and gently splash my face. I rub in a little soap and give my remaining facial hair a good scrub. Hair begins immediately raining into the sink, dusting the basin. I peer at myself in the mirror. I am now totally clean-shaven, not a hair on my face. I stare at myself for a full minute. My eyes seem bigger, and weirdly enough, I look younger. I'll have to get used to this face because I won't be wearing a beard anytime soon. It's a face that feels exposed and vulnerable.

The next morning I wake up and my eyebrows are on my pillow. I walk into the bathroom and again stare in the mirror. I am hairless. All flesh, no fur. I look like an alien. Head, face, eyebrows as white and smooth as a baby's butt. It's odd staring at myself this way. I feel as if I'm at war, engaged in battle, and this new appearance is my uniform.

It's official. I have the cancer *look*.

Shaved head, clean face, eyes glassy and sunken from heart-gripping fear and lack of sleep.

The next day, I'm in the shower and, whammo, all my pubic hair falls out. Gone. Whoosh. Swirling away down the shower drain. I'm now officially and completely hairless.

There's something about the finality of losing your pubic hair. I expected to lose my facial hair. The eyebrows were a surprise, but thinking about it for a second, losing them made sense. Looking at my face in the mirror is shocking but acceptable. I have cancer. I'm undergoing chemo. You lose your hair. Goes with the territory. I'm okay with it. I'm even okay when the hair on my arms and legs skips town. A little bit of a "Yikes!" reaction, but, again, not cause for a major freak-out.

But when the pubic hair goes?

That's a shocker. A major wake-up call. No hair anywhere else can be a style choice. Maybe I'm trying to look like Michael Stipe or Moby. Kind of cool, kind of hairless. But if you have no hair on your dick, you look sick. That's the capper. That's the signal that you're in serious trouble. Shaving a crotch can be sexy for a woman. I've seen photos in magazines.

But a guy without pubic hair? Looks like a plucked chicken.

After my third chemo session, I get slammed with a high fever, which goes nicely with the million brand-new open sores that sprout up in my mouth and throat. I can't swallow at all. When I try, it feels as if someone is drilling a hole into the back of my throat. About the only comfort I get is from chewing pieces of ice. But eating nothing but ice causes me to lose weight at an alarming rate. Dr. Mehldau checks me into the hospital for a couple of days to keep me nourished with an IV and to try to clear up the open sores.

"I swear, I haven't been near anyone's asshole," I say.

He snickers. "I believe you. But just in case, I want to keep an eye on you."

The IV takes, the sores subside, and within twenty-four hours, I'm feeling better. I'm sitting up in bed, waiting for Dr. Mehldau to check me out of the hospital, when the door opens and a man in a sport coat and tie pokes his head in. He looks like an insurance salesman.

"Mr. Schimmel, do you have a moment?"

"Jesus, I hope so. Come on in."

He bounces into the room and offers a handshake through the handles of his briefcase. "Stevie Blauner. How you doing?"

"Okay."

"Great!"

Stevie is tall and thin with a jumbo-sized head of shiny black hair that rests on his head like a dead animal. Talk about a bad wig. This guy's wearing a possum on his head that looks like it just came out of Earl Scheib.

"I'll cut right to the chase. I'm a wig salesman."

"Really?"

"Got my catalogue right in here." Stevie presents the brief-case to me as if he's offering me a box of candy.

"A wig salesman, huh?"

"Yep."

"You got one for my dick?"

"As a matter of fact, I do." He opens the briefcase with a flourish and pulls out a plastic catalogue. He starts whipping through the pages, occasionally wetting his finger with his tongue for traction.

"You gotta be kidding me," I say. "Cancer's not enough. Now I got the dick wig sales rep in my room."

"We don't call them dick wigs," Stevie says. "We call them merkins."

"Merkins, huh?"

"Yep. Merkins date back to the Elizabethan era. They're perfectly natural. They're made of real or artificial hair, your choice, and they attach with either liquid adhesive or Velcro."

"Fascinating. Do you sell a lot of these?"

"You bet. Many cancer patients are self-conscious when they lose their pubic hair so a merkin is a very sensible alternative." Stevie lowers his voice, letting me in on a secret. "It's virtually undetectable."

"Yeah? I don't have a single hair on my body and all of a sudden I've got a shrub between my legs and it's unde-tectable? You don't think someone is gonna see me naked and say, 'So, yeah, I think we should . . . what the hell?'

'What's the matter, honey, you never saw pubic hair before?'

'Not with snaps.'?"

Stevie snorts. I shrug. "Well, I guess a dick wig's better than growing three long hairs and trying to comb them over the top," I say.

"Merkin," Stevie says.

"I'm just curious. How much does one of these cost?"

"As with any product, there's a range. We have merkins starting at $44.95 all the way up to $3,000."

"For three thousand bucks, my merkin better cover my crotch and whack me off at the same time."

"I actually have a sample in my car, if you wanted to try one on," Stevie says.

"No, thanks. I'll pass."

"Okay. But if you change your mind, here's my card. I'm here at least once a week." Stevie places his business card on my night table. "Have a good day, Robert," he says.

"You, too," I say.

Stevie leaves.

"Try one on," I mumble. "Right." I pick up his card, read it, stare at it, and actually say aloud to the empty room, "This has to be a joke."

The card reads: "Wigs Unlimited" and gives a mailing address in Beaverton, Oregon.

Not a joke.

●　●　●　●　●

Sometime after my fourth session, the effects of the chemo start accumulating and begin battering me all at the same time. I feel like a crash test dummy hitting a brick wall in a Ford Focus.

First, the mouth sores. No matter how much ice I chew or asses I refuse to lick, the sores will not go away. And forget about keeping anything down. I can't get anything *in.* For three weeks straight I live on orange lozenges, Jell-O, water, and liquid Lidocaine to numb my mouth. Prisoners at Guantanamo have a better meal plan.

Once the sores start to clear up and I return to solid food, I immediately throw everything up. Oh, and did I mention the headaches and dizziness? Every room I enter is spinning like a *dreidel* (to my non-Jewish friends, that's a top). I close my eyes to get my bearings and the room spins faster. I force my eyes open to slits and try to focus on something to stop the bed from rolling, and, that's it, I'm racing into the bathroom, hunched over like a comma, praying I make it to the bowl.

All of this adds up to extreme weakness. I no longer walk. I shuffle. It feels as if there are fifty-pound weights lashed to each leg. The headaches intensify, become as relentless and incapacitating as migraines, but without the benefit of the light show. Imagine the worst rap music in the world pounding in your head, blasted at a volume beyond red line. I'm waiting for my ears to bleed.

Then, to add to the fun, *hemorrhoids.* And not just a few. A mountain range. Popping out all the way from my ass to my waist. At least that's what it feels like. Sitting on the toilet now takes all of my strength, courage, and will. I'll be honest. Taking a good shit used to bring me pleasure. It now causes teeth-clenching pain. I cry during every crap.

I see Dr. Mehldau for a once-over. In his examination room, I mentally go over my checklist of horrifying side effects, the worst of which, without a doubt, are the hemor-rhoids. They're killing me. Everything else is minor. I've got to get some relief. It's like Al Qaeda living in my asshole.

The door opens and the most gorgeous nurse I've ever seen walks in.

"You . . . you're not Dr. Mehldau," I say. *Oh, yeah. Mr. Smooth.*

"He'll be right in. I'm Meredith. I'll be doing your prelim-inary." She smiles, revealing a slight overbite.

Mannn. Would I like to bang her. Yeah, right. In my con-dition I couldn't find my dick if I had a G.P.S.

"Any side effects yet, Robert?"

"A couple," I say. "You know. A few. Minor stuff. Nothing I can't handle."

"What are they?"

I swear she just puckered her lips. She's unbelievable. She wants me. I'm all over this.

"Robert?"

"Huh? Oh yeah. Um. Well, my hair is falling out. Fell out. Everywhere. Almost. Some places still intact. A lot of virile hair still. And, okay, let's see. Oh. I have bad headaches. And I get nauseous."

"How often?"

"Let's see. Well, pretty much all the time. Pretty much always."

"Does it burn when you urinate?"

"Me? No. Not at all. Sometimes."

"Hemorrhoids?"

"Excuse me?"

"Do you have hemorrhoids?"

"No. None. Zero. Clean as a whistle."

"Wow. You're doing incredibly well. Nothing too horrible."

"Yeah. Not bad. Piece of cake. I'm very lucky."

"That's it, then. Dr. Mehldau will be right in."

She runs her tongue over her top lip, then leans over to give me a glimpse of her world-class boobs. She slowly sashays out of the room.

Call me, she whispers over her shoulder.

Okay. I'm pretty sure I made up that last part. I'm so weak and delusional that anything's possible. A few minutes later, Dr. Mehldau comes in frowning at my chart.

"No hemorrhoids yet?"

"I got hemorrhoids like you wouldn't believe. Killers. It's like there's a whole city of miniature pyramids living in my ass."

He looks up from the clipboard and stares at me, confused.

"You told Meredith you didn't have hemorrhoids."

"Have you seen Meredith?"

"I hired her."

"Then you know I can't tell her I have hemorrhoids. 'Hello, Meredith. I'm Robert. I have a horrible case of hemorrhoids. But I'm horny. Wanna screw?' I don't think so."

"Yeah. That might hurt your chances with her."

I nod. "That's what I'm saying."

He smiles and shakes his head in what to me looks like amazement.

• • • • •

I leave Dr. Mehldau armed with a prescription for pain pills, which I fill on the way home—I actually wait in the car and play with the radio while Vicki deals with the pharmacy—then as soon as she hands me the bottle, I pop them like Pez. They work quickly, dialing my pain down from the level of water torture to something more tolerable, say, getting a cavity filled without Novocain. No side effects, either. Well, one.

Constipation.

There is nothing worse than having a case of terminal hemorrhoids and being constipated at the same time. I call Dr. Mehldau. And, yes, by now I have him on speed dial. He's stuck somewhere at Mayo, his nurse says, but she suggests a laxative.

Which leads to an incident I'd rather forget.

The bottom line, no pun intended, is that I wake up in the middle of the night with a searing pain in my stomach and an overwhelming and immediate need to take a shit. I lurch into the bathroom, plop down on the toilet, and—

The next thing I hear is a siren's *warr-warr-warring.* When I manage to wake up and force my eyes open, I'm strapped onto a gurney in the back of an ambulance. Two paramedics sit on either side of me. One cups an IV drip that dangles down from a portable rod attached to the ceiling and the other jabs the needle into one of the potholes in my forearm.

"Don't tell me," I say, my voice a hazed-out slur. "I passed out taking a shit."

One of the EMTs laughs.

"Any shot we can keep that between us?"

I don't hear any response, but before I drift back off to sleep, I make a mental note that it may not be funny now, but next week I'll kill when I tell everyone about this in the infusion center.

* * * * *

Cancer beats the crap out of you. It pounds you with nonstop body shots to your ribs, chest, throat, gut, and head. You are left breathless, afraid to move, because even the slightest motion sends you reeling.

I am so weak that walking more than three steps leaves me winded, gasping for air. This actually motivates me to set a daily walking goal. I gauge the distance from my front door to the mailbox. I calculate that it's thirty feet, more or less. My goal, I decide, is to walk to the mailbox and back. Eventually.

Day one.

"Vicki, I'm gonna get the mail."

"Are you sure? It's hot out there."

"I got it. No problem."

Twenty minutes later I've made it ten feet. My lungs are burning and I'm sweating like I've just run a marathon. I turn around and inch back into the house.

Day two.

"Vicki, I'm gonna get the mail."

"Be careful."

"I will. Today's the day. I can feel it."

I get about halfway to the mailbox and then I stop, desperately trying to catch my breath. I see the mailbox in the distance, a mirage on the horizon. I vow that tomorrow's the day. Right now, I have to get back to the house before I pass out and end up back in the E.R. Man, I must be building up quite a reputation back at the ambulance shed.

Hey, you hear about Schimmel? He passed out trying to get his mail.

That's nothing. The other day he passed out taking a crap.

I just pray that I don't die from the hemorrhoids.

Day three.

I do it! I make it to the mailbox! Takes me half an hour but who cares? I squint into the mid-afternoon August Arizona sun, leaning on the mailbox, as jubilant as the heavyweight champion of the world. I take a deep breath, flip open the mailbox, and reach in.

Mail hasn't come yet.

"It's all right," I say to a cactus. "I never get anything anyway."

I call Vicki to pick me up in the car.

Day four.

Establishing a new goal.

Walking to the mailbox and *back*. Literally takes me two weeks, but I finally succeed, slapping at the front door as if I'm an Olympic gold medalist crossing the finish line. Eventually I build up my stamina so that I'm strong enough to walk to and from the mailbox twice in a row. I slap the front door each time.

Yeah, it's true. Walking to and from my mailbox becomes the highlight of my day. But it's not just making it to the mailbox. The walk itself and all that comes with it are the highlights. The soothing heat of the sun beating down on my face and neck. The smell of the desert flowers. The sound of a desert animal, a lizard maybe, swishing through the sand. The sky, cloudless and blue as a swimming pool.

Taking all this in. Taking all this in slowly, because slow is the only speed I know. But you know what cancer teaches me from these walks?

Slow is the speed at which we should live. Always.

•   •   •   •   •

At a certain point during chemo, I start to lose feeling in my fingertips. Numbness descends and my hands become, for all intents and purposes, dead. I stare at my fingers as if they're attached to someone else. I consciously tell them to move, to pick up that pen, to touch that spoon. I coax, cajole, make idle promises to my own fingers. Finally, after what seems like half an hour, they respond, moving in extra-slow motion, the fingers of a stranger.

Certain simple tasks that I'd taken for granted, such as buttoning my shirt, become difficult, if not impossible. I have to abandon my favorite pair of jeans because they have buttons on the fly instead of a zipper. If I needed to pee, I couldn't undo the buttons. The only upside to my finger numbness is that when I jerk off, it feels like somebody else is doing it.

It's crazy. The one thing I never stop thinking about is sex. No matter how weak, dizzy, nauseous, or gross I feel. Sex is always on my mind. I don't know if it's because I'm a guy or because I'm me. In my mind, I remain a virile, healthy, horny guy. Doesn't matter what's going on with my body. I can be aching all over, weak, bleary-eyed, throwing up, and have diarrhea, but if a cute woman walks by, my mind goes, *Boy, would I love to have sex with her.*

And then my body sends my brain back the following message: "Good luck, pal. She's sitting on a bench ten feet away. Have sex with her? You can't even make it over there."

Then at a certain stage my body trumps my mind. I get to the point where I'm thinking, *I'm so horny. I really need to masturbate,* but my body's voice will jump in and say, *So, what, I gotta get up, go to the bathroom, and get the lotion? You want me to go through all that right now? Screw it. It takes too much energy.* It really does.

Walking to the mailbox one day, I start making a mental list of all the things I used to take for granted that now require superhuman effort. Stuff that I do every day but never think about. Easy, no-brainer stuff. Like putting on my shoes.

One of the toughest, most exhausting activities of my life. Takes forty minutes on a good day. And when I finally pull on my shoes, I collapse in my chair, totally wasted. But I feel as if I've accomplished something incredible. What a rush. It's like I've won the Olympic gold medal.

"I did it." I grin, staring at my sneakers all laced up and ready to roll. "I got on my shoes. Wow."

Then there's the next step up. Those things that I'm afraid I'll never do again. Like driving a car. My dad's almost eighty but he once said, "I'll never give up driving. If you take away my car, you might as well cut off my dick."

I know what he means. In our culture, driving a car is a sign of virility. I don't happen to agree with that. I think getting laid in a car is a sign of virility. And getting a blow job while driving a car means you're a real guy. Probably about to be a dead guy, but a *real* dead guy.

I think about this because one day I arrive at the mailbox, flip it open, and find a letter addressed to me. Which is stunning because I never get any mail. Fingers fumbling, barely operational, I manage to rip open the envelope. Beautiful. I finally get a letter and what is it? A notice that I have to renew my driver's license. Yeah. The Schimmel Touch.

I make the trek back to the house, then after a nap, call the Department of Motor Vehicles. After only a forty-five-minute wait, I get connected to a bored customer service representative. Here's a question: why are the most bored, annoyed, angry people on the planet hired as customer service representatives? I wonder if they actually do hire the nicest people they can find and screen out the really nasty people.

Hi. I have a question?

I have an answer. Kiss my ass.

Wow. A little hostile, don't you think?

Hey, I'm one of the nice ones. You want to talk to someone who didn't make the cut?

Back to the real phone call. A woman's voice teetering on the border between annoyed and surly suddenly spits out, "Can I help you?"

"Yes. I just got a notice that I have to renew my license—"

A bored-as-hell sigh whistles through the phone. "You can't do it on the phone. You have to come down to the Department of Motor Vehicles and renew your license personally."

"See, I can't do that—"

"Then you will not be allowed to operate a motor vehicle. Do you have any further questions, sir, or may I be of assistance to somebody else?"

"Can you actually *be* of assistance to somebody? Because you haven't been of any assistance to *me.*"

"Sir, if you'd like to talk to my supervisor—"

"I have cancer." That stops her like a train. *Cancer.* Always a surefire attention getter. "I can't come down there and renew my license because my immune system's shot. I can't be around other people."

"I'm sorry. I didn't realize—"

"Unless you want to take my picture while I'm wearing a surgical mask and a ski beanie."

She actually laughs. Then her voice rises into a compassionate lilt. "You know what? Forget it. You don't have to come down here. Just don't get caught driving with an expired license. You take care, okay?"

"Thank you."

"Sorry if I was rude. I'm not usually that way."

"Well, you probably have a pretty stressful job."

"Oh *yeah.* Some people, you know?"

"Well, it takes a special kind of person to do your job. I can tell you're really patient and caring."

Okay, yeah, I know I'm blowing smoke, but what the hell? Maybe she'll be nicer to the next person.

It works. I can feel her beaming through the phone. "I don't get that a lot," she says. "You made my day."

"Hey, you made mine, too."

That part I mean.

Weird thing about cancer. Sometimes it brings out the best in people. Including me.

●   ●   ●   ●   ●

Without a doubt, cancer is the ultimate *Get Out of Jail Free* card. The first time I realized this was when Vicki was driving me to Mayo and we were late. Not her fault. Took me an extra half-hour to put on my shoes.

Vicki is normally a cautious driver. But there are no cars on the road, no cars in sight, and she's driving like she's in a parade. I'm a little on edge.

"Come on, Vicki, let's go. I'd like to get there *today*."

"Okay, fine," she says, and reluctantly presses the pedal to the metal.

Out of nowhere, a highway patrol car slides in behind us, hits the siren, and flashes us.

"Nice call," she says to me and pulls over. A large state cop saunters over to us. Vicki rolls down her window.

"What's the hurry, ma'am?"

"Officer, I know I was speeding. I'm taking my husband to chemotherapy and he's late."

"Hi, officer." I croak out a cough. I give him my pathetic, sunken-eyed look. I'm not trying for the Academy Award. It's just the way I happen to look.

"Oh, I, uh, see." The poor guy doesn't know what to say. I'm sure he feels like, *Damn. This guy looks like shit. What if he's dying, chemo's his only hope, and he misses his treatment because*

I'm writing him a speeding ticket? I might be costing him his life.
Do I want that on my head? That could send me straight to hell.

"You people go on. Take it easy, though, okay? And good luck."

"Thank you, officer," I say. Vicki smiles, waves, and pulls the car off the shoulder and back onto the highway.

"Wow. You say the word *cancer* and doors open," she says.

And I can see her mind working—

We walk into a crowded restaurant right in the middle of the dinner rush.

"Hi. Two for dinner."

"I'm sorry. There's a forty-five-minute wait."

"Forty-five minutes? My husband has cancer."

"You don't think he's gonna make it forty-five minutes?"

"It's a very aggressive cancer—"

"Shit. Okay. Right this way."

Or I hear her on the phone with the pool repair guy. "Yes, listen, the pool pump's broken."

"We can get there in about three weeks."

"Three weeks? My husband has cancer. He can't wait that long. His only joy is watching the kids swim."

Watching the kids swim? Who does she think she's married to, Henry Fonda?

Bottom line? Cancer sucks 99.99 percent of the time. But if you want your pool cleaned the next day or you want to go to the head of the buffet line, cancer rocks.

Yeah, .01 percent of the time having cancer is a real plus.

SESSION FOUR

"TRYING ANYTHING"

EMBRACE THE CANCER

"Embrace, the, cancer."

Dr. Mehldau's words.

I roll them around in my head.

Embrace the cancer.

It's a weird notion, really. Counterintuitive. I'd actually like to *kill* the cancer.

But Dr. Mehldau says bring it close, make it mine, own it.

I will. I have to. Cancer is a part of my life now. No way around it. And I'm going to do whatever it takes to get through the chemo. I want to get better. I want to beat this thing. I want to *live.*

I don't know what will work so I'll try anything. I'm open. I remember—

Montreal, 1998. I'm performing at a comedy festival. My parents are in town, visiting friends. I meet them for dinner at Gibby's, a famous steakhouse. My parents' choice. They love the place. It's a pain in the ass for me because I no longer eat red meat.

We sit down and the hostess hands us our menus. My mom pores over hers, practically licking her chops.

"Robert, you have to get a steak here. It's unbelievable."

"Ma, I don't eat red meat. You know that."

"You can make an exception tonight. Because I'm telling you, this is the best steakhouse in Canada."

"But I don't eat steak. I haven't had red meat in a really long time. Like seven years."

"That's why you don't put any weight on." She snaps her menu shut. Case closed.

"Ma, listen. I don't want it. I'm going to get the salmon. You can get the steak. Enjoy."

"I have an idea," she says. "You get the steak, *I'll* get the salmon, and if you don't like the steak, we'll switch."

"Why don't we just switch right now?"

The waiter appears. Guy in a tux. "Are you ready to order?"

"Yes, we are," my mother says, opening her menu, peering at it with adoration as if she's looking through my bar mitzvah album. "My son would like the porterhouse steak—"

I'm horrified. "*Porterhouse* steak? I can't eat that. Even if I was eating meat, there's no way I could eat that."

"Robert, it's the best of both worlds."

"What other world are you talking about?"

She lays her menu down patiently. "You get the fillet *and* you get the strip."

I lean over to her and whisper, "Ma, it's just meat. Yeah, like the bone is the border and the other part is Cabo San Lucas. It's the same thing. The bone just separates the two meat parts. The best of both worlds. Jesus."

"And how would you like that cooked?" The waiter presses on, wanting to get away from us and on with his life.

My mother tilts her head, locks her eyes into mine. I've been here before. Like a billion times. I'm not winning this battle.

"Fine. The porterhouse," I say. "Medium rare."

"Medium *rare?*" my mom says. "Are you out of your mind? God knows what could be in there. Parasites, vermin, plus the meat companies shoot those cows up with hormones and steroids, and don't forget mad cow disease."

"Those are the reasons I don't eat meat in the first place!"

Now the waiter's getting fidgety. "If you want, I can come back—"

"Stay right here," my mother says. Never let a waiter go. Her motto.

"Ma, will you please let me get the fish and you get the steak?"

My mom glances up at the waiter with puppy eyes, defeated. "Okay," she says. But she's pouting.

Our meals arrive. I take a bite of my salmon, my mom attacks her steak. She falls back into her chair in ecstasy.

"Oh *myyy,*" she moans. "You've got to taste this steak."

Now I'm begging. "Ma, I don't want to taste the steak."

"One bite. Please. One bite isn't gonna kill you. One *bite*—"

"Okay, okay, o*kay.*" There is no winning here. If I don't choke down a tiny piece of the porterhouse, we're never gonna get out of here. She triumphantly slashes a small rectangle of steak with her knife and fork, stabs it with her fork, and *choo-choos* it toward me as if I'm five.

"Open the tunnel, Robert."

"Ma, I'm almost fifty years old. Please."

"Fine. Break my heart. I only survived the Holocaust."

"Jesus." I roll my eyes, pop her fork into my mouth, taste the steak just to shut her up, and—

I can't believe it. It is beyond delicious. This is the best experience I've had in probably fifteen years. It actually rivals my first honeymoon night.

Of course, I feel terrible. I'm awash with guilt, but that lasts only a second because I ask for another taste and another and then my mother airlifts another small rectangle of steak, which I devour like it's the forbidden fruit from the Garden of Eden.

Looking back, I realize that eating that porterhouse steak in Montreal was the foundation for the attitude that will get me through my cancer treatments:

Try anything.

Something that you previously considered crazy, harmful, or forbidden just might be exactly what you need now.

And different things work for different people. You never know what will have an impact, what will be successful, what will save you.

There are no more long shots. Common sense is off the table. Everything and anything is worth a bet.

Because I have nothing to lose.

•   •   •   •   •

One of the first things I try is Reiki, a Japanese method of stress reduction and healing. A friend of mine swears by it. Says he knows a Reiki master, someone who he claims can take away the bulk of my pain and kick out most of my cancer just by laying hands on me. I'm game. What do I have to lose?

The Reiki master shows up one afternoon when I'm lying in my hospital bed, checked in because of a worrisome fever and a serious world of hurt. The master is a wispy woman who looks a lot like Elvira, Mistress of the Dark. Thin, pasty face, shlumpy floor-length sundress, plunging neckline, and a gazillion beads around her throat and wrists that keep clanging, sounding like wind chimes. Right before the Reiki treatment, she removes the beads (keeps on the dress, damn it) and starts moving her hands all over my body. I think I hear her chanting or humming or murmuring, but I can't be sure. Then she murmurs something about either giving me her energy or taking my money.

Through it all, I'm trying to allow the Reiki *in*. I want the Reiki to penetrate. I jam my eyes shut and try to go with the flow, letting her run her hands over me, Reiking me all over the place. I want this nutty shit to work. I really do. If Reiki takes away some pain, I'll become a Reiki convert and sell it in airports. I don't care. So I try. I close my eyes and surrender.

Right in the middle of my Reiki treatment, Dr. Lugo, one of the oncologists on the floor, walks in. He stops dead in his tracks. "What the hell are you doing?"

"Reiki," I mutter.

"Oh," he says. "Uh-huh."

"She's almost done," I say.

"I'll come back," he says. "Reiki on."

"He broke my rhythm," Elvira says. "You want me to start over?"

"Is it the same price?"

"Well, no, I'd have to charge you for a whole new session."

"Can't afford that. Pick up where you left off."

"Do you feel anything?"

The comic in me wants to say, "My wallet feels lighter," but I just say, "Yeah. Something. I don't know. I feel a little lightheaded."

"That's good, Robert," Elvira says. "Very positive. You can't get all the benefits of Reiki after only one treatment."

"Yeah," I say. "I figured."

Elvira steps back, assesses me with what appears to be a look of genuine surprise. "You know, a lot of people are skeptical. You have a really good attitude. Thank you."

"No," I say. "Thank you."

•   •   •   •   •

Later, after the Reiki lady leaves, Dr. Lugo comes back in, carrying with him a slightly superior air. He swivels his head toward the door as if Elvira's still standing behind him and says, "You don't really believe in that stuff, do you?"

The truth is, I don't know. Yeah, Reiki seems a little off the beaten track, that's fair to say. But just because Dr. Lugo thinks it's a bunch of mumbo jumbo doesn't mean that it doesn't exist. A lot of Western medical practitioners barely know anything about nutrition. I've often asked my doctors, "What if I eat this food and eliminate that one, will that help?" They shrug, admit ignorance. In my experience, they are, for example, much more comfortable prescribing antibiotics than touting antioxidants.

So I just say, "You know what? I'm not sure what I believe. I don't know if Reiki helps. I do know that it doesn't hurt. It's just hard for me to dismiss it and say it's baloney."

Dr. Lugo's not going to let this go. Guy's a tad intractable. "I'm just saying that in purely medical terms—"

"Here's the thing." I exhale deeply. Catch my breath. "What Reiki does for that hour while Elvira is humming and floating her hands all over my body is give me some *peace.* If that's all I get out of it, one hour of peace, then it's worth it."

"Well, okay, if that's what—"

Abruptly I sit up and, without realizing it, clamp my hand onto Lugo's wrist like a handcuff. "Dr. Lugo, you can't go twenty-four hours a day, each and every day, obsessing about your cancer. Nobody can. You need a break. It cannot be in your face nonstop. I can't continually remind myself that if this doesn't go away, I'm gonna die and I'm never gonna see my kids again. So if nothing else, Reiki distracts me. And that is worth everything."

Lugo swallows and nods. "I'm sorry."

"A lot of people believe in Reiki. I'm just saying, *What the hell? Why not?* But don't worry. I draw the line. I'm not gonna waste my time having somebody do a rain dance in my bedroom. The stuff's gotta make *some* sense."

He grins. "Well, that's good to hear."

"Yeah. Rest assured. I'm not gonna sacrifice a goat in here or anything."

I release his wrist and fall back onto the bed. "She was kind of cute, the Reiki lady, in a stoned-out-sixties-acid-flashback-mushroom-eating sort of way," I say.

"I guess so. I wasn't born until 1970."

"You're a child."

"Yeah. I got a lot to learn."

I drift off to sleep.

. . . . .

And so begins a series of alternative, sometimes far-out *distractions.*

I try acupuncture. I go to a Chinese woman in Phoenix who asks me to lie down on a table covered with what feels like butcher paper, then sticks about a thousand little needles into my legs, arms, stomach, ears, neck, and one in the middle of my forehead, the unicorn. She turns off the lights, fires up a couple of incense-burning candles, and puts on a Yanni CD.

"See you soon," she says and leaves the room.

Immediately my thoughts turn dark, resting in that place I try to avoid, the place where all I can see and say is, *I'm gonna die if this shit doesn't work. Never gonna see my kids, never gonna see my parents, never gonna—*

And then she's back. "How you doing?"

"Okay." She begins pulling the needles out and I manage a peek at the clock. Over an hour has gone by. "*What?* Are you kidding? You were gone for an *hour?*"

"Yes. You were sleeping real good. Sorry I have to wake you up."

This may not sound like much, but between the throwing up and the worrying about dying, I don't get a lot of sleep. It turns out that acupuncture is more than a distraction.

It's a gift.

. . . . .

I have less success with meditation. I try various deep-breathing exercises from yoga. Nothing works. My mind sails off into thoughts of death, darkness, and despair, resulting in horrifying bouts with the Big A, anxiety.

My parents want me to keep trying. Both are devotees of Transcendental Meditation and have been for years. They try to teach me how to block out everything in my mind and find nothingness. I close my eyes, focus on the color blue, and—nothing. I can't do it. I'm a TM failure.

"Ma, it's not working."

"Try again, honey. It's so worth it. Believe me."

"I'm sure it is. But I'm just not one of those people. I can't clear my mind."

My mother looks around the room furtively, as if she's a spy.

"Okay, look, I'm not really supposed to do this," she says, "but I'm gonna give you my mantra."

"Your mantra? Ma, I'm so touched."

"You can't tell anybody because, well, you know—"

She looks around again, peeks over her shoulder.

"Why do you keep looking around like that? You think there's secret mantra police? 'Hey, where'd you get that mantra? That sounds an awful lot like the stolen mantra we gave your mom.'"

"This is serious, Robert."

"What do think I'm gonna do, sell your mantra on eBay? I promise, it's safe with me."

"I trust you," she says. "Okay. Here." She whispers her mantra into my ear. She steps back and gives me a knowing little nod. I nod back and mouth, "Thank you."

And then I try meditating using my mom's mantra.

Nothing. I just can't block anything out. The next day I say to her, "It didn't work. Your mantra."

"You're kidding. I don't believe it. It never fails."

"Well, for you. For me, no."

"I'm so disappointed."

"Yeah, me, too. So, okay, how do I give it back?"

"You can keep it. I got another one."

"Really? That's so weird. I feel like we're talking about a jacket."

Of all the conversations I've had with my mother, this one is by far the strangest.

•   •   •   •   •

What does work, surprisingly, is guided meditation, also known as visualization. A friend tells me about a series of natural healing CDs that Dr. Andrew Weil has put out. Dr. Weil talks about the value of taking a cleansing breath, then following that by visualizing something that you really, really want. Which in my case is to live.

Dr. Weil himself narrates the CDs in his soothing baritone, managing to sound urgent and folksy at the same time. He makes you *want* to listen and then makes you feel as if the information he has to impart is vital. I'm hooked. After getting the breathing down, I try a visualization, guided by his voice, following his instructions.

"Close your eyes. Picture this. You're down by the beach, and the ocean's crashing onto the sand, and you can smell the salt in the air—"

I'm pulled in by his words and caught up in the picture that I paint in my mind. I am swept up and carried away. For the next hour I'm gone, sunk into the sand by that beach, lost, out of my head and cocooned away, far from my worries and my cancer, as close to being physically transported to some exotic location as I could possibly be without leaving my room.

When I come back from my hour at the beach, I feel relaxed, soothed, lightheaded. I start thinking, *Being at the beach felt so real. But it wasn't real. It was all in my head.* So, then, what is reality? Isn't the world you create in your mind reality, *your* reality? Do things really look the way they do? Or do we *create* things to look the way we want them? That's called perception. Man, I am *tripping.*

I do visualization every day. For me, it's necessary. It amounts to a mini mind trip, a mental vacation. I always come back calmer, refreshed, and armed with new insight. My attitude shifts. I honestly feel that I am a lucky guy. The cancer has obviously upended me, thrown me for a loop, but it has also opened me up to so much that I could never have seen before.

I begin to reorder my priorities. I see that all my relationships are shifting and deepening, and I accept that. And my perception of life changes. I don't look at cancer as a punishment for what I have done or not done in my life. Cancer just *is.* As crazy as it sounds, if I get through the chemo and kill the cancer, I will be grateful to it.

• • • • •

Vicki suggests that I try crystal therapy. She knows someone whose cousin is like the third-best crystal therapist in the Southwest.

"What do I have to do?" I ask Vicki.

"That's the best part. Nothing. She comes to you. She brings everything, candles, music, and the crystals, of course. This could be very good for you, Robert. It's all about connecting to your inner place of healing."

"I don't know. I'm open to almost anything, but this sounds wacky."

"It's not. Crystal therapy goes back thousands of years, to the ancient Hindus. Oh, one thing. She's really booked up so the only time I could schedule her is tomorrow at two, and that's when you're supposed to be at the clinic."

"Yeah, no problem. Let's cancel my appointment at the clinic so I can spend the afternoon with some crazy lady and her rock collection. Like I would ever do that."

So the next day at two I'm lying in bed with candles burning on my nightstand, while Inez, a woman in sandals and a flowing floral robe, hovers over me, her fists closed and bulging with crystals, Yanni singing from her portable CD player.

By the way, I'm pretty sure I've discovered the cure for cancer.

Yanni.

If I beat this thing, it's because the cancer cells couldn't stand Yanni anymore. They packed up and got the hell out of my body as fast as they could so they wouldn't have to listen to any more of that music.

"How you doing, Robert?" Inez speaks in a superhigh voice loaded with sympathy. Her voice is birdlike. She chirps.

"Fine. Doing great."

"That's wonderful. Okay. What we're going to do is locate your seven chakras. You know what a chakra is?"

"An ice cream flavor?"

Inez chirps, "Not quite. Your seven chakras are the areas in your body that need to be aligned and in balance to promote health and healing. They're your meditative spots. Including, by the way, your third eye. Your disease blocks your chakras, clogs them up, so to speak. The crystals, specifically the one you choose, will help in the unclogging, alignment, and balancing. Understand?"

I don't have the vaguest idea what she's talking about. "Got it," I say.

"Great. Robert, you're very spiritual." Chirp, chirp, chirp. "Okay, now close your eyes."

I do. I smell a whiff of strawberry wafting over from the candles. Behind me, Yanni's yowling as if he's got somebody's thumb up his ass.

"Now, I want you to hold out your hands. At the same time, I'm going to hold out a selection of crystals. With your eyes closed, pick one."

"What am I feeling for?"

"The right one. For you." She pauses. "I don't have to say anything more. You'll just know."

I shrug and close my eyes. I wonder how this would look to Dr. Lugo if he walked in now. Not sure I'd be able to explain the crystal lady to him. I might just go with, *Okay, doc, here's the truth. I'm an easy mark.*

"Robert," Inez tweets, "the main thing is to clear your mind. Don't think. *Feel.*"

I nod and reach out my hand. My fingers fumble through the crystals in Inez's hand, four or five cool, smooth, jagged little torpedoes. I touch each of them, and then I feel my fingers involuntarily closing around one near the hook of her thumb.

"This one," I say. "Yeah. This is the one."

"*Per*fect," Inez trills.

I open my eyes and observe the pale blue stone pressed into my palm.

"You've chosen kyanite," she says. "Kyanite is the absolute best stone for aligning the chakras. And it helps you communicate with your spirit guides and angels."

"Sounds like I'm already dead."

"Not quite," Inez says.

"Just curious," I say, rolling my crystal around in my fingers. "How much does one of these cost? Roughly."

"The kyanite is one of your less expensive stones. The top price is only about eighty dollars. Then, of course, you can always add a setting, for a ring, say, or a necklace, and that'll drive the price up. I actually brought a catalogue. We sell the stones, and accessories as well."

"Eighty bucks, huh? Seems like a bargain for something that allows me to communicate with my spirit guide."

"I *know*. Good thing you didn't choose amethyst. Those can run you over two thousand dollars." Inez laughs. Then shifts into a tone that's all business. "Okay, Robert, I want you to lie down, close your eyes, hold your kyanite stone to your chest, and try to focus only on your crystal. Concentrate on it. Give it your full attention. Can you do that?"

"I'll try."

"I'll guide you through it," Inez says.

I happily go with her. She, too, chooses to send me off on a sandy beach under a soft, soothing blue sky. Fine by me. I love the ocean. I feel connected to it. In fact, I make a promise to myself right then, an instant before I drift off to the melodic sounds of Inez's chirping.

If I make it through this, I'm going to buy a house on the beach and I'm going to live there for a year, no matter what it costs. I don't care if I have to sell my car and everything else I own. I'm going to do it. I owe it to myself. And I'm not going to put it off, because one thing I've learned, you never know what the future holds. You have to give yourself permission to live life to its fullest. Living on the beach. That's the one thing I have to do.

Later I find out what it actually costs to live on the beach, and I say, "You know, living three blocks away isn't that bad."

But for now, I'm gone, lost in the spell of Inez's chirpy voice, in the smell of the strawberry candles, even in meowing Yanni, because I know that while crystal therapy will not cure my cancer, it, too, like Reiki and acupuncture and all the rest, takes me on an hour vacation from the horror of the chemo and the madness that surrounds it. And that's why I believe in it.

●　●　●　●　●

I start keeping a journal.

I get the idea from Nadine, the nurse at the infusion center.

As usual, I've brought in muffins and doughnuts for the staff to share. Nadine tears the top off a blueberry muffin and pops bite-sized pieces into her mouth.

"You have an unbelievable attitude," she says, and then gives me a wonderful compliment. "We all look forward to seeing you. You brighten up the day."

"Thank you. That's very nice. I try. Some days are easier than others."

Nadine pours a cup of coffee from a silver thermos she keeps handy. "Have you thought about keeping a journal?"

I'm intrigued. "What would I write?"

"I'm talking about an Oprah kind of thing. You wake up in the morning and you think of something good. Start your day that way. Write something positive."

"You mean, instead of, 'Well, good morning, I'm up, and damn, I've got cancer, I'm dying, and if the chemo doesn't work, I'm finished?'"

Nadine smiles. "Yeah. Instead of that. Be honest. But look for something good."

I look at her, and now I smile. "A journal, huh? Why not? I'll try anything."

● ● ● ● ●

I cover all my bases. I buy both a reporter's notebook and several packs of three-by-five index cards. My idea is to write one positive thought per card. Frankly, I buy the index cards as a safety measure. What if I open up my reporter's notebook and I have no positive thoughts? The blank pages will stare at me, depress me. Somehow the index cards are less intimidating. I needn't have worried. The thoughts pour out of me unchecked, uncensored, unedited. I write until my fingers ache. The thoughts help me focus and keep me sane. I keep the cards with me. I read what I've written at various times during the day. I shuffle the cards, read them in a different order, find new meaning. In the course of my chemotherapy, I will write thoughts on hundreds of index cards. Here are just a few:

- *Learn to embrace my cancer. It is mine. I do not belong to it. Cancer might be a part of my life, but it doesn't rule my life.*
- *Every time my children smile at me, it feels as though God is smiling at me.*
- *I don't want to die scared.*
- *Beggars can't be choosers. Yes, they can. They chose to be beggars.*
- *To get closer to God, you have to get closer to yourself.*
- *Are guys with big dicks ever concerned about their size?*
- *I have to be a proactive parent.*
- *Tune everything out for a few minutes a day and find peace of mind.*
- *Fight negativity!*
- *It's hard to take everything with a grain of salt when you're on a sodium-restricted diet.*
- *Make today the most important day of your life.*
- *Maybe when we hit a low tide emotionally, we need to look for all the good things about life, ourselves, our inner beauty.*
- *People come up to me and ask, "Why don't I ever see you on TV?" I tell them, "It's probably because I'm not on."*

●   ●   ●   ●   ●

I change my relationship to food.

It begins with this card I write: *Eat healthy. Appreciate your food and don't rush through meals.*

I buy a couple of books by Dr. Weil. I read them both in two days. His books are full of wisdom and insight and connect with me deeply. Among other things, I'm struck by his suggestion that you should make a ritual out of eating. Seems like we're always in such a hurry. It's tremendously unhealthy to sit down at the table, shovel the food into your mouth, and race toward your next activity as if the world's going to end if you don't take that phone call right then.

Take your time. Look at your food. Really look at it. And if you're cooking, enjoy and experience each moment of the process, including picking out the food that you're going to eat. Examine the tomato that you're about to slice up and put into your salad. Smell and touch the lettuce you'll be using. Cooking is very tactile. And, I discover, very sensual. Also, when you slow down, cooking becomes almost a form of meditation.

I create a sort of mantra. I write on an index card: *This food is good for me. It's filled with vitamins and minerals and will nourish me. No more junk food.*

I really get into my food. I see everything, especially fruits and vegetables, in a whole new light. I'm awestruck by an orange—the shape, the color, the touch, the smell. I hold it close to my nose, take it in, and, I swear, I imagine the orange grove. I even imagine the seed from which the orange grew. I picture the soil with just a seedling popping through the dirt, then the rains come and the seedling grows into a tree and the fruit swells and ripens. I feel connected to all of that. I don't feel alone. And I don't feel separate. I feel part of *life*.

· · · · ·

Ray, a friend of my brother's who I know casually, calls me up after I'm diagnosed. Ray is a nervous, ferret-faced guy who spent most of high school camped out in the corner of my brother's room getting high and listening to Canned Heat and Pink Floyd. He speaks in a high-pitched nasally voice that sounds like a dentist's drill.

"Hey, man, I heard. I'm really sorry."

"Yeah. Thanks, man," I say.

"What a ream job," Ray says. "You know, with the show and all."

"Yeah."

"Are you sick yet?"

"Oh yeah."

"What are you doing for the nausea?"

"Basically, throwing up."

"I hear you, man."

"My doctor says I can smoke pot."

Ray brightens. "Really?"

"Yeah. He says pot helps with the nausea."

"I can get you some pot, man," Ray says.

"I don't think so, Ray."

"I'm talking about some really good pot. Not the crap they sell in Compton, man. I'm talking about some serious West Side, rock star weed."

"I don't want it, man. But thanks."

Ray's dental whine revs up into ultrahigh speed. "Robert, please. Don't deprive me of this. I want to do this for you."

"I don't really smoke pot."

"But if it helps with the nausea, why not try it? Why *not*, man?"

"I don't know—"

"Robert, I'm begging you. I want to do this for you. I didn't know what I could do. Now I know. Please. I just want to do this for you. Please let me do this for you. *Please*."

I feel as if Ray's whiny voice is about to drill through my skull. At this point I'll say anything to shut him up.

"Okay, fine. I'll try it."

"Oh, man, thank you *so* much. This really means a lot to me. I just want to help you, man."

"Thanks."

Ray arrives at my house early that evening. I answer the door and Ray bounds in. He throws his arms around me in a wrestler's clinch, intermittently massaging my back in slow circles as if he's kneading pizza dough. I'm unsure if and when he will release me. Finally I break his clinch. Ray nods solemnly.

"Robert," he says. "Man," and bear hugs me again, nearly breaking a rib.

He pulls away, wipes at a tear that's trickled down to his chin, and slaps his right coat pocket. "Got the goods."

I lead Ray into my room. This whole evening is rapidly turning bizarre. It's as if I've never left high school and I'm sneaking Ray in to smoke grass while my parents are waiting for me to join them at the seder table. Although in this case I've sneaked Ray in under Vicki's nose while she's in the shower. I close the door behind him.

"You don't know what this means to me," Ray says. He pulls out of his pocket a small, folded-over plastic Baggie a quarter filled with pot and presses it into my hand. "Here, man."

"Thanks, Ray."

"That'll be sixty-five dollars," he says.

I stare at him. "What?"

"That's how much it costs."

"I'm not giving you any money. I didn't want it in the first place."

"You're gonna stiff me? That is cold."

Ray inhales massively and crouches into a catcher's stance. He seems frozen there, injured, betrayed. Now it appears that I have two choices: pay him or take the chance that he will stay locked in that position forever as if he were a potted plant.

"Jesus, Ray." I grab my wallet and fish out four twenties. Ray whisks them out of my hand like a train conductor.

"I don't have change, man," he says whippet fast, pocketing the bills. "I'll put the difference toward your next bag."

I wave him away. I'd like nothing better than for him to leave so that I can flush the contents of the Baggie down the toilet and crawl into bed alone with my spiritual self-help books and my nausea.

"So let's get high, man," Rays says, popping up out of his crouch and cracking his knuckles so loudly I cringe. He reaches into another coat pocket and produces a pack of rolling papers. "Pass me the pot."

"What are you doing?"

"Rolling a joint."

This doesn't feel right. First, I don't even want to smoke a joint. Second, I definitely don't want to share a joint with Ray. I've started chemotherapy, my resistance is low, and while I haven't discussed this with Dr. Mehldau, I'm pretty sure he'd advise me against sharing a marijuana cigarette with a drug dealer.

Ray finishes rolling the joint. He licks both ends, holds the cigarette up to his nose, and takes a long slow whiff. "Man, this shit is fine. Let's fire this baby *up.*"

From a pocket *inside* his coat (the guy's got more pockets than Coco the Clown) he produces a plastic cigarette lighter. With a magician's flourish, he flicks the lighter's top, releasing a violent blue *broosh* that would make a blowtorch proud, nearly searing my eyebrows. Ray leans into the flame. He catches the joint's fat end, inhales a mighty chestful, holds it in for an agonizingly long thirty seconds, then exhales a thick brown cloud that hovers Hiroshima-like over my bed.

"Oh *yeahhhh.*" He's grinning goofily, high already. "Come on, Bob, baby, let 'er rip." Ray offers the joint to me, forbidden fruit. I take it, study the thing, then in what feels like slow motion, bring it up to my lips.

It's been forever since I smoked a joint. Can't even remember the last time. At least twenty years. Even then I was never a get-high-and-blast-Metallica type of pot smoker. Pot has the opposite effect on me. *Had.* I smoked grass and the world slowwwwed down. The world became ice cream and cotton candy. All the colors of the rainbow. Fluffy whipped cream clouds dancing. Candy cane striped poles instead of lampposts. Calliopes. Merry-go-rounds. Happiness all around.

"Imagine me and you, I do, I think about you day and night, it's only right—"

Yeah. The Turtles. Forget Pink Floyd. Can Canned Heat. My getting-stoned soundtrack belongs to the Turtles. Hey, who doesn't love the Turtles?

"So happy togetherrrr. And how is the weatherrrr?"

Oh, I'm high. I'm so high. I'm so fucking high. I'M SO FUCKING HIGH. I'M SO . . . *AHHHHH!!*

I'm shaking. My pulse is pounding in my head. I'm burning up. Sweat pours off my forehead into my eyes, temporarily blinding me. My hands are quivering out of control. Tremors. I have tremors. I'm shivering. And I can't breathe. Voices are screaming in my head. They won't shut up. I can't breathe. I'm suffocating! I'M SUFFOCATING!!!

I hear Vicki's voice, far away, a distant echo. "Robert, what's the matter?"

"I don't know. These voices in my head. Maybe the pot was sprayed with something."

My mother now, hand to her mouth. "Oh, God, he's never going to be the same."

"Ma? Are you here? The doctor said I could smoke pot, remember? I was just following doctor's orders."

"Robert, can you hear me?" Vicki gripping my arm.

"Hey, man, it's not the pot." Ray's offended. "That stuff's sweet. Mrs. Schimmel, have a taste. Seriously. Try some."

"It's not the pot," I echo. "I'm having an anxiety attack."

"That makes sense," Ray says. "Because it's definitely *not* the pot. You're absolutely having a panic attack. Makes total sense. You have cancer, you could die, what's it all about, Alfie? These thoughts have to fuck you up, man."

"Ray, not now, please," I say, pressing my thumbs into my forehead.

"I'm just sayin'."

"You are really stoned, Robert," Vicki says. "*Really* stoned."

"Yeah," I say. "No shit."

"You have to come down," my mom says. "You want a Xanax? I think I have one in my purse."

"Yeah," I say. "A Xanax would be good."

My mother rustles through her purse, which contains countless cold remedies and an array of prescription bottles, one of which does contain Xanax. CVS pharmacy carries less medication. Why she has Xanax in her purse and how she knows it will sober me up are questions I don't want to deal with, but I pop the pill, chase it with half a bottle of Evian, and fold myself into the living room couch. Vicki escorts Ray to a back bedroom where he'll sleep off his high. Later she'll call a friend or maybe animal rescue to retrieve him.

The Xanax does the trick. The pot high wears off, the Turtles fade away, and then, suddenly, a cliché—I get a huge case of the munchies. I head into the kitchen and swing open the refrigerator. Nothing but carrot juice, soy milk, broccoli, cabbage, cauliflower, caraway seeds, and a bunch of other useless, healthy food. I squat down to the freezer, yank that open, rummage through the shelves, and finally find pay dirt: three unopened boxes of ice cream sandwiches. I pull them out, stack them up, rip them open, and polish off two and half of the boxes standing over the sink.

Two days later, in Dr. Mehldau's office, with him at my side, I step onto the scale for a second time. He shakes his head. "Amazing. You've actually gained two pounds."

"Wow," I say.

"And you had vomiting, right?"

"Record-breaking pukage. You would've been proud."

"Well, right now you're a medical miracle. You go on chemo and you *gain* weight. What's your secret?"

"No secret. I just did what you said. I smoked a joint and ate a shitload of ice cream."

"Be careful," Dr. Mehldau says, his eyes widening. "That could lead to the hard stuff." He ticks them off on his fingers: "Cakes, pies, doughnuts, muffins, cupcakes . . ."

Big cartoon laugh at his own joke.

* * * * *

You cannot fight cancer alone. This I know. To that end, I surround myself with people who are not afraid to talk about what they're going through. You have to talk about it. Otherwise you give the disease power over you.

I once spoke to a guy named Ted who told me that he didn't know where I got the strength to make fun of cancer. I corrected him.

"I'm not making fun of cancer," I said. "I find comedy in some of the experiences I've had, but I do not think cancer itself is funny."

"I have cancer," Ted said. "I'm terrified all the time."

"So am I. But I try to live in each moment, take each day as it comes. Today was a good day. I feel pretty good right now. That's all I got. Today."

"I just can't get over the fear," Ted said.

"You have to talk to somebody about that."

"I can't," Ted said. "I don't want to talk to anybody."

"You're talking to me right now. That's a start."

In the end, I'm not sure how much I got through to Ted. My heart goes out to him and people like him who never get out of the denial stage. If you don't talk about it, then you're running from something that just *is*. You can't deny it; you can't outrun it. And I've found that the best people to talk to are those who are either in the same boat as you or have gone through it and survived. We all have to be realistic. But to beat cancer, you need to remove as much negativity as possible.

I think of Magic Johnson. He was diagnosed with HIV in 1992. Sixteen years later, he's still opening up shopping malls and movie theaters and barbecue places all over Los Angeles. He's a testimony to not giving up. It's a fight. As Michael Landon said, "If I don't beat cancer, I'll die trying."

Unfortunately, he lost his battle. I'm going for a different ending.

• • • • •

Finally, I laugh. Remembering what Norman Cousins said about the healing power of humor and seeing how people in

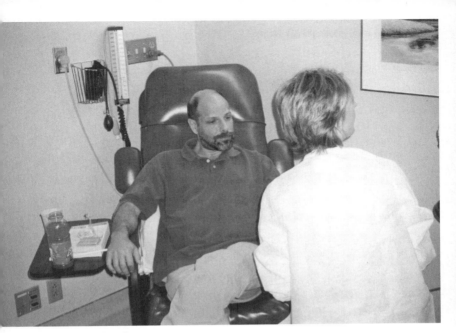

urse Jody giving me my first chemo.

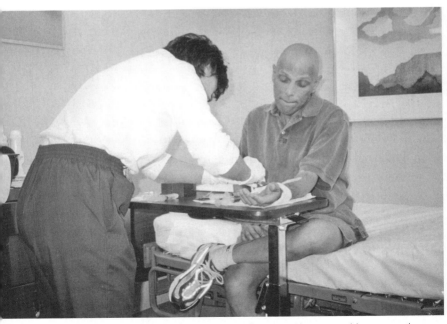

r the third treatment. You can already see the changes. Jody is now a brunette and has put on about nty pounds.

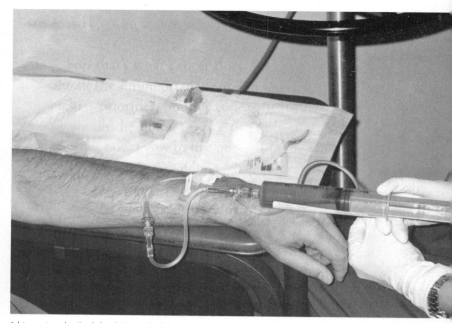

Adriamycin, aka "red death." I asked the nurse why she was wearing thick rubber gloves, and she said, "I c[an't] get this on my skin. It's toxic." And I thought, "Toxic? But you're injecting it right into my vein!"

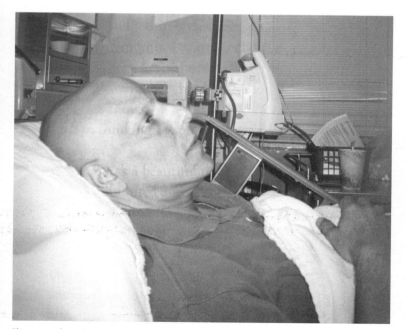

That's me after I found out what my co-pay was.

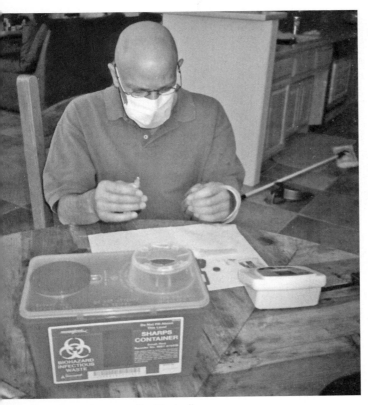

ng Neupogen shots to boost my white blood cells.

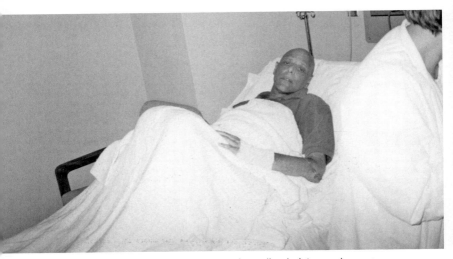

e's me after getting my testicle removed. As you can see, the swelling hadn't gone down yet.

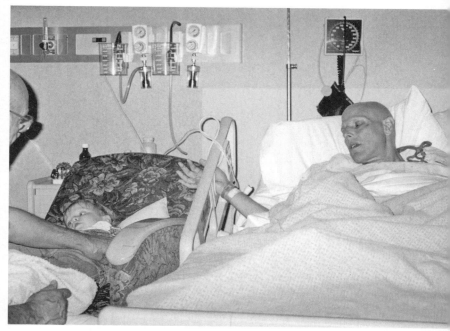

My dad, Jacob, and me, with one more treatment to go.

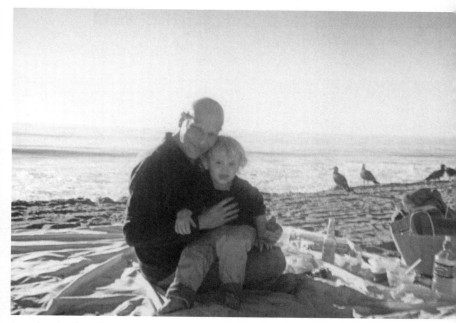

At my favorite place, the beach, with Jacob after my last chemo.

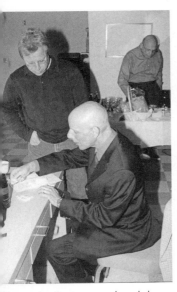

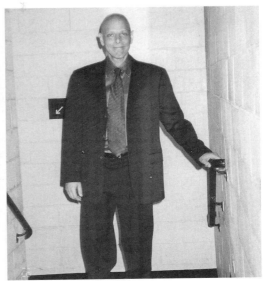

...manager, Lee Kernis; me; and my dad
...stage at the Monte Carlo.

On my way to the stage at the Monte Carlo.

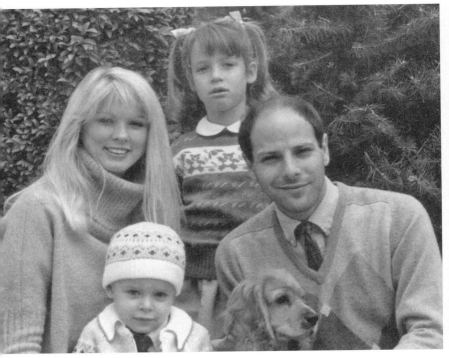

...i, Derek, Jessica, and me.

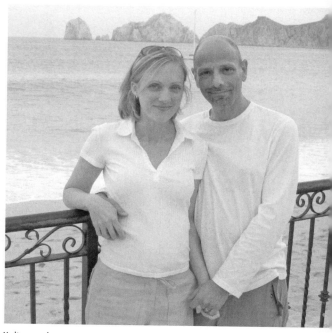

Melissa and me.

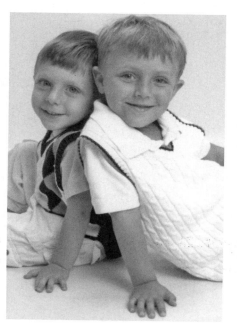

Max and Sam.

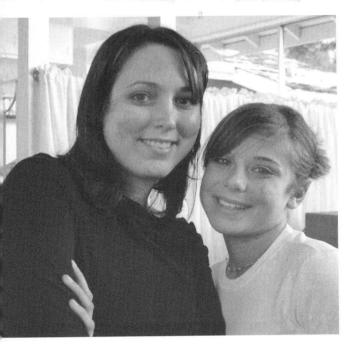

ca and Aliyah.

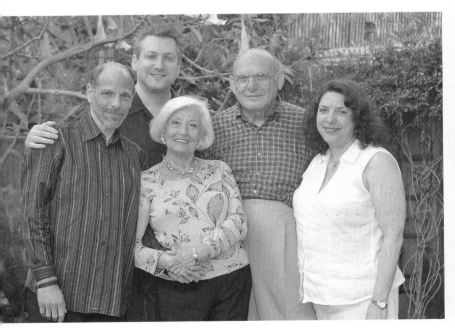

my brother, Jeffrey; my mom and dad; and my sister, Sandy.

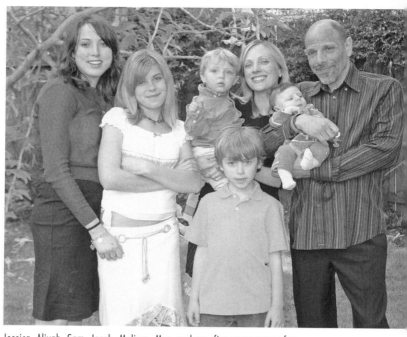

Jessica, Aliyah, Sam, Jacob, Melissa, Max, and me, five years cancer-free.

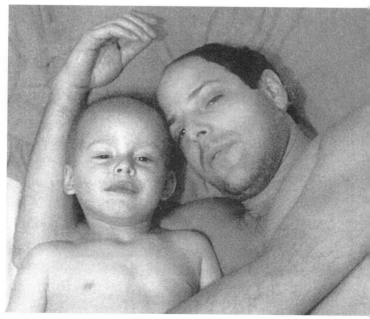

Derek and me.

the infusion center react when I tell them a joke leads me to seek out distraction in comedy. I get my hands on all the comedy albums I can find, starting with Steve Martin, Don Rickles, and Bill Cosby. When friends ask me what they can do for me, I tell them to send me comedy albums and DVDs. I listen to Lenny Bruce, Redd Foxx, Bill Hicks, Sam Kinison, Andrew Dice Clay, Bob Newhart, and Phyllis Diller. I watch Bill Maher, Dennis Miller, the Three Stooges, the Marx Brothers, Jerry Lewis, and Mel Brooks.

I bring my albums into the hospital and share them with the people in my support group. I watch them get lost in their own laughter and I am inspired. I want to be part of their recovery; I want to help them feel *good,* even for a short time.

Because when you're laughing, there is no other emotion in that moment except for joy. No anger, no depression, no fear. Just joy. Making somebody who is sick laugh seems to me to be the most important and fulfilling thing I can do.

I know what's going through their minds. The worst, scariest shit you can imagine is playing nonstop: *My life is over* or *What did I do to deserve this?* or *How will I get through this?* and, most of all, *Am I dying?* I want to take them away from those thoughts. For in the moment that they laughed, in that one moment, they weren't sick, and they weren't afraid.

•   •   •   •   •

Cancer and I share a long and checkered history. We go back forty years, when I was diagnosed with a potentially precancerous, undescended testicle. That story's coming up.

But on December 2, 1992, I was inducted into an exclusive society: the Fucking Unlucky Club. On that day my son Derek died from brain cancer. He was eleven years old.

People often called Derek an old soul. I agree. There was no doubt that there was something timeless about him, as if he'd been here before and was just passing through in order to deliver a message. And to change lives. He was an incredible teacher. I learned so much from him, not necessarily from the words he spoke, but from the way he acted, especially when he was at his sickest.

Despite his body being weak and frail from being ravaged by cancer, Derek was the strongest, most determined person I've ever met. I'm sure he didn't seem that way at first, when you saw him lying in his bed attached to a million tubes. We fed him through a tube in his stomach and he lived with an IV that went straight into his heart. Many days he breathed inside an oxygen tent. I can't imagine his physical discomfort, but he never complained and lived his life more fully than any healthy person I've ever known. He made every second count. He was full of grace and pride and humor.

He laughed, all the time. Man, did he laugh. He gave me the gift of being my most receptive audience. Sometimes I'd just look at him and he'd remember something stupid I'd said or something silly I'd done and he'd break up. He taught me to appreciate what I have and to live now, in the moment. My son Derek, age 11, cancer victim, taught me how to live.

Of course, it took me eight years, until I had my own cancer, to fully *get* Derek's life lessons. Better late than never.

Here's one example of Derek's spirit.

He had just turned eleven and had had a couple of very good days. I'd just bought a brand-new Toyota Land Cruiser and wanted to show it off to him. Still had on the dealer plates. "Paper plates," Derek called them.

It was a beautiful, warm afternoon and I sat on the edge of his bed, hanging out. I suddenly had this crazy idea.

"Hey, Derek," I said. "You wanna go four-wheeling in the desert? We'll take the new Land Cruiser."

"Are you kidding? Sure."

I leaned in and said just loud enough for the hospice nurse to hear, "I'll even let you drive."

The hospice nurse, a bull of a woman named Lana, said, "No way I'm gonna let you do that. You cannot take him four-wheeling in the desert. God knows what will happen to him out there."

"What's gonna happen out there that can't happen here?"

Lana started to object again, but I wasn't listening. I piled Derek, his IV machine, and his oxygen tent into the Land Cruiser and we headed out into the desert. In Arizona, you can drive down a main highway and if you pull off the road, you're right in the middle of the desert. Which is what I did. I pulled off of Scottsdale Road, turned onto Bell, and veered into a vast open patch of desert sand. The landscape shimmered in the heat. Here and there a cactus stood tall, a prickly sentry. Perfect spot for Derek's first driving lesson.

"Okay, buddy," I said. "You can drive."

I sat Derek in my lap. He squirmed around, got comfortable, then stretched his legs down and made sure he could reach the pedals. Finally, he settled in.

"Ready?"

He nodded.

"Okay. Try not to get us killed."

He pressed his sneaker onto the accelerator. We jerked about five feet in the air, plopped down in the sand, and swerved to the right. Derek spun the steering wheel and straightened us out. His face lit up.

"You're doing great, Derek. Just watch out for that—"

Cactus.

Crunch. Derek sideswiped it, bounced off, smacked into another plump cactus, scraped the shit out of that, then scratched a boulder that suddenly appeared in front of us like a mirage. I gripped the door handle. My knuckles turned white as paper, and then Derek whipped the wheel around to avoid another oncoming cactus, which he managed to only graze. He swung the steering wheel violently. I honestly thought we were going to tip over.

I looked at Derek. He was in his own world, engulfed in sheer bliss. I could see it in his smile, a smile I'd never seen before, a smile that was all joy, and as we pounded the crap out of another cactus, and the bumper of the brand-new Land Cruiser fell off, all I could think was, *Why didn't I rent a car?*

• • • • •

Derek is always with me—his memory, his spirit, his energy. I take him with me onstage. I can feel him. And as I battle through my own cancer, I know that in some way Derek has prepared me for it. Maybe I've inherited his spirit and his attitude and that is what's driving me now. I know kids are supposed to inherit traits from their parents, not vice versa, but as I said, Derek was an old soul, traveling through, and maybe, just maybe, in my hallucinations or in my dreams or in my meditations, Derek used to be my father. No, I'm not flipping out. Cancer makes you see things in a whole new light if you let it. It's one of the benefits. Call me crazy or call me enlightened, call it religion, call it mythology, or call it *Star Wars,* I don't care. With cancer, you have to be open to anything.

SESSION FIVE

"GETTING LAID"

SEX DURING CHEMOTHERAPY

Lying in bed after an exhausting hour of vomiting, I manage to open my eyes into slits and stare at the ceiling. As the room starts rotating again and I slam my eyes shut, I have a random and disturbing thought:

Am I ever gonna get laid again?

This is followed by a series of rapid-fire and recurring questions:

Am I gonna die without ever having another orgasm? Was the last orgasm I had the last one I'll ever have? When was the last orgasm I had? Was it that time I got laid or that time I masturbated? Did I have my last orgasm looking at photos of Jessica Alba in Us *magazine? Is that fair? Don't I deserve more?*

To me, getting laid—or at least feeling as if I *want* to get laid—means that I'm alive. If I'm horny, I'm still here. Sometimes you just need to know that the mechanism works, that the blood flow from the station, your brain, is going to arrive on time at its destination, your dick. More than once, actually many times, I have been lying in my hospital bed, an orderly wheels in a female patient, I look over at her, and say to myself, *Boy, I'd love to jump all over her.*

I have no idea what she's here for. She could have AIDS, hepatitis C, syphilis, *and* gonorrhea: the STD combo plate. I don't care. She's female, she's breathing, and I'm horny. Good. I'm still ticking.

Feeling horny is life-affirming. It's really that simple. There is the obvious connection between creation and continuation. *Life.* When you go through chemo, you are always monitoring yourself. Lost my hair, puking my guts out, weak as hell, can barely stand up, but suddenly the *Sports Illustrated Swimsuit Model Special* is on TV and, whoa-whoa-whoa-yeah-yeah-yeah, I'm horny. Soon as your dick stops working, then you worry.

It does happen. Especially to guys with prostate cancer who have their prostates removed. Most of them can't get it up. It must be horrible. You see a pretty woman and you say, *Wow. Look at her.*

And your dick says, *What?*

Over there. Look. Her. The one with the big tits.

What are tits?

That would kill me.

• • • • •

Sex is on the mind of the oncologists, too, because one day Nadine comes into my hospital room and hands me a booklet called *Sex During Chemotherapy.*

"I thought you might want to look at this," she says.

"Thanks," I say and read the title. "Does everyone get this or just me?"

"Everyone. But we figured you'd appreciate it the most."

"Yeah. Does this come with an instructional DVD?"

Nadine laughs.

"That's actually not a bad idea," I say. "I'll be the instructor."

Nadine laughs again, a little too much in my opinion, then points to the pamphlet. "Let me know if you pick up any tips."

"I'm only gonna read the good parts. Hey, some of these pages are stuck together. Those must be the good parts."

She's gone, but I hear her laughing down the hall.

I open the pamphlet and begin reading: "Treatments for cancer can cause discomfort, fatigue, and intense pain. *Hey, is this about cancer or divorce?* Still, it's possible to be sexual throughout treatment, just differently than before. Self-pleasure through masturbation is easiest because you set the pace."

I look up. *Set the pace? I usually don't last long enough to have a pace.* I skim the rest of the booklet and toss it onto my nightstand.

I think about my own experience with sex during chemotherapy. I'll sum it up in one word: none. But there are other general truths. For example, nobody in my support group wants to die. Everybody wants to be cured or in re-mission. And everybody wonders if they will ever have sex again. Especially the guys. We are deathly afraid that we will never be able to get it up again. It's an overriding, debilitat-ing fear. We fear the doctor coming into our room one day and saying, "I have good news and bad news. The cancer is gone, but so is your sex drive."

Most guys would say, "Wait a minute. Can't I have a little cancer and still be able to have sex?"

Because without sex, where does that leave us? Spending the rest of our lives photographing butterflies and picking up seashells? It's just a matter of time before you go home and swallow every pill in your medicine cabinet.

Guys are essentially insecure. Even healthy guys. It's because women control sex. If a woman who looked like the hunchback of Notre Dame walked into a roomful of guys and said, "Okay, am I gonna get laid tonight or what?" there'd be bottles and glasses breaking as guys trampled over each other to get to her. But if a guy walked into a roomful of women and said, "Am I gonna get laid tonight or what?" the women would say, "Hey, asshole, get outta here." They would. Trust me. At least that's what they said to me.

Guys will do anything to keep the sex drive going, to keep ourselves operational. I've talked to some of the guys in my support group and they've told me about various devices that are on the market to help them get it up, during and after chemo. This is serious stuff.

First, there's your average, everyday penis pump.

The one nine out of ten doctors recommend is the plain old suction tube type, the kind you stick your dick in, and then pump up. Similar to a penis-enlarger pump. So I'm told. Apparently once you're comfortably in place in the cylinder, all you do is press the handy dandy squeeze bulb apparatus, which then increases the blood flow. You pump, you squeeze, the blood flows, your dick grows, hello porn star.

Personally, this scares me. I really wouldn't want to experiment with increasing blood flow to my penis. I envision a very unhappy ending involving an exploding penis and a front-page story in the *National Enquirer:* "Comedian Robert Schimmel Blows Up Own Penis After Losing Sitcom Deal."

The second most popular penis pump (I can't believe I just wrote those words) involves inserting an actual pump in the fleshy region near your balls. It's like having a permanent balloon in your dick. I'm not sure why this version is so popular (it doesn't get my vote), but the idea is, when you want to have sex, you pump yourself up with the valve next to your balls and the balloon inflates. How long it takes to *de*flate is a question I might ask. And does it give you that funny falsetto voice like when you're loaded at a party and you suck the helium out of a balloon to impress some girl?

I keep trying to get my mind around this method. You're getting it on, things are happening fast, getting hot and heavy, and you have to stop and say, "Hold on, honey, be right with you."

Vroosh, vroosh, vroooosh.

"Wait a minute. What is that?"

"Nothing, nothing. Just a valve near my balls that operates a balloon in my dick. It'll only take me a couple of minutes to blow it up. Unless you want to. Hey, where are you going?"

Then there's the most foolproof penis implement of all.

The dick rod.

There's probably a more technical name for it but I don't know it. The dick rod consists of a six-inch piece of hard rubber, like rebar, that a doctor surgically implants into your penis. Once it's in, you have a miracle dick. You can bend it, twist it, tie it in a knot. It's like Flubber. So, basically, you're walking around, going about your daily life, running errands, doing whatever it is you do, and if you get home and you want to have sex, wham, you whip out your dick, and bend it any way you—or she—wants. It's great. It's like a gooseneck lamp. You can swing it over your head, play cowboys and cowgirls, *yeeha,* whatever. And even if you can't come, your dick stays hard forever. You can keep on going and going until she finally says, "I smell burning rubber, do you?"

We talk about this—penis pumps, dick implants, sex during chemo, masturbating, merkins, all of it—in the support group. Fortunately, I don't have the need for anything artificial. Although if I couldn't get it up, I wouldn't rule it out. If it takes a pulley for me to get an erection, so be it.

What's interesting is that we also talk about how God fits into sex.

We all pray. We pray to be whole, to be right, to be back the way we were. Even those who have lost their faith either before or since being diagnosed talk to God. We have time on our hands and we spend a lot of that time alone. We feel different. We are different.

A few weeks ago, I'm sitting on a bench in the mall. Although there are five hundred people around me, I feel completely alone. Nobody knows me; nobody acknowledges me. I watch the people who pass me and I think, *They're all walking by me, laughing, talking, shopping, living normal lives. And I could be dying right now.*

I stand up and walk among them and I am invisible. I feel like a ghost.

And so we pray.

Please God, I don't want to die. Please allow me to get through this. I'll be a better person, a better father, I promise. Just please let me live.

That seems natural. But what about praying during sex or when you're masturbating? Is that natural? Somehow it doesn't seem right. Seems like a waste of prayer. It seems so normal, though, to make sure everything is in proper working order. Unfortunately, you can't fool God. You can't hide. You can't beat off under a blanket or in a closet because He can see what you're doing.

I don't know. Maybe I'm wrong. Maybe it's perfectly acceptable to ask God for your dick to work.

If you come, is that a sign? And then do you take the next step and pray for sex?

Or in my case, do I go for broke and pray for my other testicle to grow back?

• • • • •

I had my first brush with cancer when I was thirteen. As I said, I was born with an undescended testicle. My left one. The doctors wanted to perform experimental surgery on me, which involved pulling my ball down. I've blocked out most of the details, but essentially they had to open my ball sac, stitch it to my thigh, hook my left ball to a kind of bungee cord, then yank on it. Basically, we're talking ball-stretching surgery. They were concerned that an undescended testicle could be an indicator of cancer later in life. Okay, they got that right. Unfortunately, they didn't get the surgery so right because apparently after they pulled my ball down and unhooked it, it shot right back up. Like the ball hitting the bottom bumper in a pinball machine. Makes me very glad I was unconscious during the procedure.

About fifteen years later, I'm having a routine physical. My internist, call him Dr. Stern, has a kind, round face and is incredibly short, about as tall as a jockey. We're in the last leg of the exam when Dr. Stern asks me to drop my boxers. He wriggles his hand into a pair of rubber gloves and starts examining my scrotum. He suddenly frowns. "Your left testicle feels funny," he says.

"Well, I've had an undescended testicle," I explain. "Ever since I was a little kid."

I cough. It's not that easy having a conversation with a guy while he's cupping your nuts. At least not for me.

"It feels funny," he says again, still clutching my left ball. I wonder if I should offer to buy him a drink. Then Dr. Stern moves his hand over to my right ball and squeezes. This I don't like. I grunt.

"Yeah," he says. "That's what I thought. Your left testicle hasn't developed the way it should have."

Oh yeah. That's just what you want to hear during a routine checkup.

"*Your left ball hasn't developed the way it should have.*"

Great. I have one normal ball and one pygmy ball. Wonderful. My ego is doing cartwheels.

"I want to do a biopsy," Dr. Stern says.

"Really?"

"A precaution. But I think we need to do it."

"Okay, so, what, you stick a needle in there and you—?"

"No," he says.

"No?"

"A needle? Who told you that?"

"Nobody. I just assumed—"

"No needle. We take your testicle out, we do the biopsy, and then we get the results."

"How do you put it back?"

"We don't."

"You don't put my ball back?"

"No. What for?"

"What *for*? Because it's mine. I want my ball back."

"Doesn't work that way."

"I'm only gonna have one ball for the rest of my *life*?"

"Robert, a lot of people are walking around with only one ball."

"Yeah? Like who?"

Dr. Stern scrunches up his forehead. Thinks. "Bruce Lee," he says finally.

"Bruce Lee?"

"Yeah."

"He's not walking around. He's dead."

"All right. Bad example. There are a lot of guys, believe me. Lot of macho guys, too."

"You mean unlike me."

"Let me think for a minute." Dr. Stern drops his chin onto his hand, rests it there, and studies the floor. "Okay. Yeah. He has one ball."

"Who?"

"That tough-guy actor. You know who I mean."

I take a shot. "Charles Bronson?"

"Yes. I think so."

"He's dead, too. Jesus."

"Well, if you're interested," Dr. Stern says, "I can put a fake one in there."

"I don't want a fake ball."

"No one will know the difference."

"Really?"

"Let me get one. I'll show you. You can hold it. Play around with it. Tell me what you think." He shuffles toward a metal file cabinet.

"Play around with it? What is it, a toy?"

Dr. Stern unlocks one of the file drawers and rummages around inside. "Here we go," he says, pulling something out of an envelope.

He leans his back into the file drawer, closing it with a clang, and shuffles back toward me. He hands me a small flesh-colored rubber sphere.

"This?" I say.

"Yep."

The "ball" looks nothing like a ball. It looks like a novelty item you'd buy at Halloween, one of those funny pink faces with two exaggerated wide eyes, floppy ears, and goofy grin. I stare at Dr. Stern.

"You think this looks like a real ball?"

"Once it's in."

I roll it around between my palms. I squeeze it. I smush it. "Feels weird."

He shrugs.

"No offense, but you can definitely tell the difference," I say.

He shrugs again. "Think about it."

I do. I think about it very carefully. First, there's no way I could ever jerk off again without saying to myself, *Yeah-yeah-yeah. Man, my left ball just doesn't feel real.* I certainly couldn't do the blindfold test with myself, the which-is-my-fake-ball? test. It's clear which is real and which is Rubbermaid.

Second, what about getting laid? If a woman touches you for the first time and says, "Wow, your left ball feels funny," you feel tempted to ask her, "Really? How many balls have you held that make you an expert? Great. I'm sleeping with the country's leading fake ball authority."

Once you get past that, how do you explain it?

"Robert, what's this?"

"What?"

"This. Your left ball is weird."

"Oh. Okay, you know what? It's not real."

"It's not *real*?"

"Yeah, see this one's real, this one isn't. I lost that ball. I didn't *lose* it per se. They had to take it out. So I had a fake one put in. See, I didn't want just one ball. I'm insecure enough. Hey, why are you getting dressed?"

Maybe some guys wouldn't mention it at all. I just feel compelled to bring it up. Full disclosure. I think it's best to get it over with early, before foreplay, somewhere between the hot and heavy kissing and the tearing off of the clothes.

"Look, I gotta tell you, before we go any further, I have a fake ball."

It sounds so bad. Feels like it's gonna put a damper on the whole evening, ruin the romance. I'm probably paranoid. Because, come to think of it, I don't think I've ever heard a woman talk about balls. Either in real life or in a porno movie. I've never heard, "Hey, Greg's got some really nice balls."

You don't hear that much. The only time women talk about balls is when a guy has only one, a fake one, or three.

I'm also a little worried about my reputation. Women talk. Word gets around. I can see myself walking into a party and everybody whispering and pointing, *buzz-buzz-buzz,* "Look, it's Johnny One-Ball," "Hey, Bob, you wanna play *ball?*" "Hey, you didn't see a *ball* around here, did you?"

Who needs that?

I consider all of this, but finally I decide to go for it. Then right before the operation, Dr. Stern drops another bombshell.

"The material the prosthetic testicle is made from has a kind of thermos bottle quality to it. You follow?"

"I think so. My fake ball is like a lunch pail. Is that what you're trying to say?"

"Sort of. What I'm saying is that it will adapt to outside temperatures."

"Give me an example."

Dr. Stern scratches the top of his head. "Let's say you're outside in the snow, sledding, or skiing, or something."

"Sledding? Do I look Swedish?"

"Just go with me. When you come inside, into a warm house, your body temperature will increase, but your artificial testicle will remain the temperature it is outside."

"Wow. And the other way around, too, right? So if I come out of a hot bath and get into bed with a woman, she's gonna say, 'This is weird. Your body is cool but your left ball is hot.'"

"Exactly."

"Yeah. Quite a conversation piece, this fake ball. Dr. Stern, I don't know about this."

"Robert, it's no big deal."

"Not for you."

Dr. Stern grins and then jabs me in the arm with a needle, injecting me with a little something to take the edge off. Otherwise, if I spend one more second thinking about what is about to happen in my very precious lower region, if I contemplate that Dr. Stern is about to remove my left testicle and replace it with a heat-and-cold-attracting circular piece of flesh-colored plastic rubber fake ball, I just might back out.

Within seconds I'm floating, gonzo, feeling no pain, stoned, giddy, all my anxiety evaporated, except for one last tiny remnant, an image of a gorgeous nurse tonguing into my ear, "I've always found you so sexy, Robert. Unfortunately, I only go for guys with two balls."

And then I'm blinking into the blinding overhead lights of the operating room, and through a squint see Dr. Stern, round-faced, barely tall enough to perform the operation without a ladder, smiling up at me.

"You want to see it before we put it in?" he says.

"Yeah. I would."

"Okay." He turns to a nurse a few feet behind him. "Give me one of those prosthetic testicles, would you?"

"Here you go," she says and tosses it to him. My future fake left ball arcs toward Dr. Stern, hits him right in the hands, and pops out.

"Lost it in the lights," he says, stooping down and scooping it off the floor. He looks at it, frowns. "This one's too big."

The nurse shrugs. "It's the smallest one they make."

"You know what?" I say. "Fuck you guys."

By now, Dr. Stern, the nurse, and the rest of the blue-scrubbed operating support staff are roaring.

"A little pre-op humor," Dr. Stern says, catching his breath. "Come on, Robert. We'd only do this with you."

"That's great. You really had me going. You guys have a lot of fun in here, don't you?"

"Oh yeah," Dr. Stern says. "We have a *ball.*"

He holds for a second, then they all burst out laughing again. Ha-ha-ha-ha. I feel like I'm in an *SNL* take-off of a medical show, the unfortunate guest star about to go under the knife.

• • • • •

The good news is that I don't have testicular cancer. As for my fake ball, Dr. Stern is right on the money. Nobody notices that I have one regular ball and one made of Silly Putty. The question never comes up.

Except years later when I go in for an MRI.

I'm about to lay down inside the torpedo-shaped, claustrophobic capsule, which I'm actually looking forward to because it's the only place I can get any peace and quiet, when the nurse steps in. What a nurse. She looks like Scarlett Johansson, only hotter.

"Hi, I'm Lulu."

"Nurse Lulu. How you doin'? I'm Patient Robert."

"I can't believe this. I'm such a big fan. Do you think later, maybe, I could—"

Give you head?

Wait, did I say that out loud?

"—have your autograph?"

"Sure. Absolutely. You bet. Definitely."

Man, is she hot.

"Ohmygod. That is *so* cool. Thank you *so* much. Okay, before we begin the scan, I have to ask you a couple of questions. The answer is probably no, but are you wearing dentures or do you have any prosthetic devices?"

Do I really have to tell her about my fake ball?

To make matters worse, Nurse Lulu tee-hees in a super-sexy voice.

I don't want to tell this hottie who I'm fantasizing about that I have one nut. What a turn-off. That'll really kill my chances with her. But I don't want to go inside the MRI tube and have the machine go *whirrrr-whirrrr-whirrrr* before it blows up, and then have Dr. Stern's voice come over the loudspeaker like the voice of God, thundering at me, "Bob, you didn't lie about the ball, did you?"

I have to tell her. But maybe I can save the day by making up something cool about how I got it. Something exotic. Something that will help me get laid, instead of turning me into a carnival freak.

For a while I considered having the procedure done in Vietnam so I could tell everyone that I lost my ball in Nam. Think of the edge that'd give me. Women would assume I was a war hero.

Poor guy. He lost his ball in battle. But he says with a little bit of sex and the occasional good one-ball massage, he has a chance to overcome the memories of war. It's my patriotic duty to take care of him. Do my part for the vets.

I couldn't go through with it. Before I slide into the MRI machine, I tell Nurse Lulu the truth.

She doesn't bat an eye. Doesn't faze her at all.

Since then, so far, so good. Nobody's asked about the fake ball during sex. Nobody seems to care. Or maybe during those three minutes of passion, nobody noticed.

SESSION SIX

"GIVING UP"

TWENTY-ONE WEEKS

In my cancer support group, which consists of a dozen people who are on the brink of facing death, we mainly talk about life. We talk about our families, our passions, and, believe it or not, our futures. One by one we speak about what we have done and not done. We talk about our loves, losses, and regrets. We talk about wishes unfulfilled and plans unmade. We make promises to each other and ourselves, promises that include a tomorrow that sees us living in it. We vow to remove all the bullshit from our lives and to get our priorities in order. We give ourselves permission to live our lives to the fullest, now and forever.

I believe in all of this for all of us. It is exactly how we should have been living our lives *before* we got diagnosed.

Because you never know. You cannot predict *what* will happen to you *when*. We expect our lives to work smoothly, to keep clicking like clockwork. We take so much for granted. We shouldn't.

Remember Siegfried and Roy's show and the trick where Roy stuck his head inside a white tiger's mouth? They performed the trick a million times without incident. It became routine, almost automatic. But one night, the tiger looked at Roy and said, "This shit stops *tonight,* motherfucker." You know the rest. Cancer taught me you can't take anything for granted.

It starts with attitude. I honestly said, "Okay, how many treatments do I have? Eight? That's it? Eight and then I can go back on the road? When do I start?"

My motivation begins with Derek. I saw what he went through and I saw his attitude. He was a fighter to the end. Part of what motivates me is that I want to beat the thing that took Derek. I want a rematch. This time I'm gonna win.

It gets harder and harder. As my treatments progress and I get thinner and weaker and sicker, I rely on my will to get me through. At one point I sit at my desk and think about all the things that I want to live for. I take out my index cards and start writing a list. On the first card, I write: *I know it's not over. I know I can still make people laugh. I want to go back on the road. Cancer cannot take that away from me.*

But then I undergo treatment seven, which obliterates everything I just said.

Treatment seven teaches me perhaps the most important lesson of all:

I am human.

●   ●   ●   ●   ●

One more treatment to go. One more. Just one more. And then—

I am lying in bed. I'm cold. So *cold.*

Suddenly, I can't breathe. My chest thumps with pain. I'm shaking. I grab the sides of my sweatshirt with both hands to try to keep them steady.

• • • • •

Where am I?

At home? In the hospital? I don't know where I am.

I am in a room. I've never been here before. The room is dark and cold and damp. I shiver.

I am standing now. I take one step and bump into something hard and solid. I squint and see that I am standing in a sea of boxes. Large rectangular wooden boxes. I rub my hand on the top of one of the boxes. The wood feels smooth and lacquered and smells faintly of cherry.

I turn around and bump into another box, and another. I am trapped, walled in. There is no escape. I can't move. What is this place? Then I realize what these boxes are.

Coffins.

Two men in suits materialize. One, Mort, sits on the edge of a coffin. He wears a black suit and flashy red tie. He seems very happy. The other man is Otto, my father. He paces between two butterscotch-colored caskets. He rubs the same casket I rubbed moments ago. Mort smiles in approval. "That's a beauty."

"How much?" my father asks.

"Eleven thousand," Mort says.

"Eleven *grand*?" My father turns to me. "Is he out of his mind?"

"Who's it for?" I ask.

"You, Bob."

I nod. Of course.

"Eleven grand's a little much for me," I say. "A little rich for my blood."

My dad tips his head toward Mort, whose legs dangle off the side of the casket as if he's five years old.

"Eleven grand for a wooden box," my dad says, shaking his head.

"That you're only gonna use once," I point out.

"This is, what," my dad says, massaging the top of the coffin as if he's polishing it, "about eighty bucks in wood and twenty dollars in hardware?"

"Dad, they're not gonna let you go to Home Depot and build your own coffin," I say.

My dad eyes Mort. "I have to say, eleven thousand dollars is a little more than I wanted to throw into a hole in the ground."

"That's cheap," Mort says, suddenly dismounting from the casket. He approaches a gold-handled coffin that's suspended above the others on a museum-style glass stand. "This one's sixty-five thousand."

"Sixty-five thousand dollars?" my dad says. "You can get buried in a BMW for sixty-five thousand dollars."

"Sixty-five grand," I say. "That's not for the dead guy. That's show business. That's so people can come to the funeral and say, 'Wow. What a casket. Come on, let's go, I have a lunch.'"

My dad nods. "You're right. They're only gonna see it for a few minutes and they're never coming back."

"Why not just rent it?" I say. "You can rig it up so that when everybody leaves, you pull a lever, the bottom opens, and I'll just fall into the hole. Then you can return the casket and get your deposit back."

"I don't want to deal with this anymore," my dad says to Mort. "We'll just take the eleven-thousand-dollar one."

"Excellent choice," Mort says.

"Yeah. Excellent choice," I say. "It's like we just ordered the entrée special."

"You want a pillow with that?" Mort asks.

"Does it cost extra?" my dad asks. "Or for eleven grand, do you throw it in?"

"I have to charge you," Mort says. "Sorry. There's my cost, labor, overhead, you know how it goes, Otto."

"Man. Everything's a la carte at the funeral parlor," I say.

"He doesn't need a pillow," my dad says.

"Are you sure?" Mort asks.

"He's not going to know if there's a pillow in there. He's *dead*. He didn't ask for a pillow when we dropped him taking him out of the car."

"I'm just thinking of the comfort level, that's all," Mort says.

"Maybe he has a point," I say. "What if I'm stuck in an awkward position for all eternity?"

Suddenly, I see a beautiful rainbow arching across the sky and I hear a symphony of trumpets, and then Jesus, in all his glory, floats down to earth, and all of the dead people rise.

Except me.

Because I can't get out of the coffin.

"Come on, Robert, let's go," Jesus says.

"I'm trying to, but my back is out. My father wouldn't spring for the pillow—"

• • • • •

I'm cold. So cold.

Seven treatments. One more. Just one more.

Vomit rises into my throat, wet, sour, violent. I squeeze my eyes shut to will it away. My head pounds with searing pain. It feels as if someone is crushing my skull between two concrete blocks. The bones in my back and neck burn.

And yet I am so *cold.*

I look down at the lump below me in my bed, my body. It feels detached, freezing, the arms and legs of a distant cadaver. I move one leg slightly and feel the layer of thermal underwear beneath my pajamas pressing against my skin, and then I feel the weight of three blankets on top of me.

Still I am so cold.

I start to shiver. My fingers shake with tremors. I need more warmth, a sweater, a jacket, another blanket, but I can't move. I turn my head slowly and focus on the closet door a few steps away. I have to get there. I lift my right leg one inch. Pain shoots through me. Forget the closet. It might as well be in another state.

I'm crashing. I want to scream. But no one will hear me. I am alone. Vicki is away, a family emergency. *Robert, will you be all right for an hour or two?*

An hour or two.

I guess I forgot that my life now is defined not by hours but by minutes. An hour or two could be the rest of my life.

My teeth start to chatter and the vomit rolls into my mouth again. I don't know what to do. I am *freezing* . . .

I hear a car pull up outside. The car door slams. Vicki? The front door of the house opens and closes and footsteps approach. The door to my room opens tentatively.

"Robert? Hey."

Steve. My daughter Jessica's boyfriend. I twist my head toward him. My teeth are clattering like the plastic ones you buy at Halloween.

"Are you okay? You don't look so good."

"Steve, actually, I'm feeling, pretty, shitty."

Each word is an ordeal. The sentence nearly does me in. I have to catch my breath before I can speak again.

"I'm so cold. I need my winter coat. In the closet."

"Winter coat? Robert, it's a hundred and fourteen out. No lie."

With every ounce of strength I can find, I force my head up and lean on my elbows. Within seconds, I am doubled over in pain.

"Steve, I need a big favor. You have to take me to the hospital."

I try to move another inch but the pain shooting through my arms and head is too much. I fall back onto my pillow.

"Steve. Please."

"Okay," Steve says. "I'm gonna lift you out of bed, slowly. Ready?"

He leans over behind me and cradles me, then with both arms brings me up to a sitting position. I weigh less than a hundred and twenty pounds, and he is barely winded. But the move leaves me gasping. Before I can catch my breath, he lifts me out of bed, places my feet gently onto the floor, swings my arm over his shoulder, and walks me to the closet.

"Lean on me. We're going to find your coat."

Somehow, some way, Steve locates my down ski jacket, then slips my arms through. He finds a wool ski hat in a pocket and pulls it over my head. Like a wounded soldier, I allow him to virtually carry me to the car. Finally, we are in his Honda, this bizarre couple, the well-muscled young man in tank top, shorts, and flip-flops, and the fifty-year-old wraith in a wool ski hat, winter coat, gloves, and pajamas snug over thermal underwear.

"Steve," I say. "Would you turn on the heat?"

"The *heat*?"

"Please. I'm freezing."

He glances at me. My entire body is shaking. I am one massive tremor. I peek at him. He is scared, poor kid, even more than I am. And I'm terrified.

"Sure, Robert," Steve says. "Anything you want."

I nod, clasp my arms around my chest. I'm ice. "Full blast," I croak.

Steve flips the temperature dial over to the red line and hits the gas. I jam my hands under my legs to keep them from shaking.

"Thanks, Steve," I spit out between tremors.

"No worries." With the back of his hand, he swabs the pond of sweat collecting above his eyebrows, his eyes trained on the highway heading through the glimmering Arizona desert to the Mayo Clinic.

And then it's like an episode of *ER*.

A sea of green—doctors, nurses, attendants—descends on me. I'm slid onto a gurney, then wheeled into a room. Voices bounce off walls, firm, professional, urgent: "White blood count zero point five," and then another voice (Dr. Mehldau?) adds, "Neutroponic fever" and "Isolation."

When I'm semicoherent, I will learn that my previously compromised immune system has shut down, clobbered by the chemo, and become essentially nonexistent. I cannot be exposed to any bacteria. The slightest infection can kill me.

I'm brought by elevator to the cancer ward. I wait in the hall while a nurse sterilizes my hospital room with disinfectant. The room is without windowsills, shelves, tables—any surface that can collect dust. I have one connection to the outside world, a large plate glass window through which I can see my children.

Miraculously, they are there now—Jessica, 22, Aliyah, 10, and Jacob, 2. They are my reason to live. When they are not here, I conjure them. I bask in their imaginary faces, the glow of their smiles. I need them to keep me alive.

I try to wave to them, but it takes too much strength. I talk to them silently. I mouth that I love them and pray that they can somehow hear me.

Then they are gone, replaced by a team of doctors and nurses who scrub themselves viciously as if they have lice, and then they wriggle into space suits, and put on gloves, and masks. They look as if they are about to tamper with radiation or take a walk on the moon. Instead, they take my pulse and give me my shots. The nurses cover me with blankets, two, three, and then a fourth, and Nadine lies down on top of me. I'm so sick I'm not even turned on.

And I feel no warmer. I'm still shaking, and now, suddenly, I'm hit with an overall ache, as if I've taken repeated body blows from Mike Tyson.

"My kids," I say in a low moan. "Can I see my kids?"

A pause, then, "Soon," a reed-thin promise from a distant, disconnected voice.

$$\bullet \quad \bullet \quad \bullet \quad \bullet \quad \bullet$$

I'm dead to the world.

While I'm asleep, Dr. Mehldau meets with my parents. He tells them that I will have to be in the hospital for a minimum of ten days. That is, if I live through the night.

I wake up twelve hours later in a different room, hooked up to multiple IVs and monitors. My body feels pummeled and bruised.

I blink at the ceiling and I start thinking about my attitude, about where I am, and about how to go on. Since my diagnosis, I have done everything within my power, everything Dr. Mehldau and the other oncologists have asked. I have entertained at the infusion center and at my support group. I have preached keeping a positive attitude. I have been *up* the whole time.

And now I have been sucker punched. Never saw it coming. I have been knocked down. Nobody is a bigger fan of having a positive attitude than I am. *Yes, you can. You have to believe. You can overcome anything.*

Well, *yes, you can* has at this instant been replaced by *no, you can't.* Because sometimes you just *can't.* There are practical issues. And there are fantasy and reality. You can't be fooled into thinking that anything is possible armed with only a positive attitude. That may be the definition of insanity.

I can't say, *If I believe enough, I can go out to the parking lot, flap my wings, and fly home.*

Everything is not possible.

Even with a positive attitude, I could die.

If the treatment doesn't work, you're dead.

And if the treatment does work, the cancer could come back. I will never be cured. The best I can hope for is remission.

The way I feel right now, this minute, I could die. Right now. I really could.

I think I will die.

I'm beaten.

What was I thinking? Did I really believe this was going to be easy? I get zapped eight times and, then, voila, it's over, congratulations, cured? Yeah. Piece of cake. Gotta have the right attitude, that's all. Upbeat. Positive. The life of the party. *Hey, did you hear the one about the dick wig salesman, ha-ha-ha, you're a riot, Robert.*

Bullshit. All of it. You can't beat this disease with *attitude.* What did I think, I'm a tough New Yorker and cancer's a rube from Iowa?

I can't move a muscle. I try to wiggle my fingers and they sting, they *sting* with pain. I want to scream, but I can't. My voice is clogged in my throat.

It's over, folks. Done. I'm fucking *done.* You want the truth? I give up. I cannot get through one more second of this. I admit it. I can't help it.

I have lost.

"Robert?"

I blink once.

"Robert?"

My dad. He stands next to my bed, but he looks far away and very small.

"How you doing?"

I swallow. "Shitty, Dad." My throat feels as if it's going to tear open. "This is really bad, Dad. Really bad."

"Bob, you've got one more treatment and then that's it."

His voice is gentle, a soft plea.

"You know what? I don't care anymore." My voice sounds hollow, as if it's being piped into my head through a tinny speaker.

"Bob—"

Again, I say, "This feels really bad, Dad," and then the words rush out: "I can't—I can't—I don't want to feel like this anymore, Dad. Right now, this moment, I don't see the light at the end of the tunnel. I don't see it. This is really, really bad. Everything hurts so much. I feel so weak—"

"One more treatment, Bob, that's all." My dad fades even farther away. He seems helpless, out of arguments, out of fight, drifting far, far away.

"Dad, I can't." And I start to cry. The tears slide down my cheeks. I sniffle, take as deep a breath as I can, and then I feel weirdly calm.

"If I'm going to die, I want it to be on my terms. Not this way. Not. Like this." I wait to make sure my father hears me. I can feel his breath dusting my cheek. His eyes are locked into mine. "Dad, I want you to unhook me. I want you to pull out all these needles and plugs."

He says nothing. I lean closer to him and I whisper, "And then I want you to take me to the window. Because I'm going to jump."

My dad stammers. "J-Jump? To where?"

"Down to the street."

"Robert—what—what would that accomplish?"

I sniff. "That way *I* decide when I'm going to die and how. And if I do it this way, I take the cancer with me. The second I hit the sidewalk, it dies with me. It can't crawl out of my body and get someone else. I take it *with* me. I kill my fucking cancer. I want to jump, Dad. Please. Open the window."

His lips start to quiver. And then my dad suddenly starts to cry. He coughs, wipes his nose with the sleeve of his shirt. He backs up two steps and turns toward the door. I reach for him, grab nothing but air. "Where you going?"

"I'll be back," he says.

I close my eyes and I sigh. My chest heaves and fills me with an ache that rattles my teeth. *Jesus. God. I'm through. I really am. I can't do this anymore. I can't.*

And then I'm aware of movement at the door. I turn my head slightly and see my dad standing in the doorway with my children, Aliyah and Jacob. He holds their hands. He hesitates half a second, and then he brings them a step closer to me.

"Tell them," he says, his voice a low hiss.

My bottom lip flutters. I am shaking all over.

"Tell them what you told me," my father says.

I look at them, my children, my reason—Aliyah, innocent, wide-eyed beauty, and Jacob, a baby, pure, too young to know disappointment and sin, both of them made purely of promise and hope and love, and I can't speak.

And then, as I look at them, I see Derek in their faces, in their eyes, and I can see his light, and I can feel his fight, and suddenly I hear his laughter, even at the end, and I remember sitting with him on the edge of his bed and telling him stories, among them my version of "Goldilocks and the Three Bears"—

"So, yeah, the Papa Bear comes down for breakfast and he says to his wife, Mama Bear, 'I'm hungry. What's for breakfast?'"

"And the Mama Bear says, 'Oatmeal.'"

"And the Papa Bear says, 'Oatmeal? You gotta be shitting me. How about bacon and eggs, or some sausage, something like that? I don't want any fucking oatmeal.'"

"And the Mama Bear says, 'Where the hell am I supposed to get bacon and eggs?'"

"And the Papa Bear says, 'The same place you got the oatmeal from, you dumb shit.'"

By now Derek is laughing hysterically, practically falling off the bed. What other dad would talk to his eleven-year-old son like that? He knows I'm insane. And he loves it. From that moment on, all I have to do is sit on his bed, put on my Papa Bear voice, and say, "I'm hungry," and he bursts out laughing.

I look now at Aliyah and Jacob and I understand, finally, completely, that this cancer is not about me. It's about them. It's about my children. I have a responsibility. I have to get through this for Jessica and Aliyah and Jacob, and for Derek. We have very few choices in life, and choosing cancer isn't one of mine. The disease chose *me*. I can only choose to give in to it or to keep fighting. And I can choose not to kill myself.

I lift my eyes from my children to my father. His eyes are moist and his mouth is trembling slightly. He stares at me silently.

When he was a child, he lost his parents. And now he is facing losing a child. I know what that feels like.

I can't do that to him or to my mother. They have suffered enough.

And then I remember a story my father once told me, the story of his survival, the story of *his* life—

•   •   •   •   •

In single file, hundreds of Jews march alongside the Nazi soldiers. All of the Jews are skeletons. Most can barely walk. A few give up right there, suddenly breaking from the line. With their last ounce of strength, they streak toward the barbed wire fence and impale themselves on it. Others simply step out of the line and stop. The soldiers respond by shooting them.

Otto Schimmel, 15, moves slowly, almost imperceptibly, baby step by baby step. The Nazis jab their captives, including Otto, with their bayonets and tell them to pick up the pace. A boy Otto's age drifts out of line, falls to his knees, sobbing, holding his hands above his head in surrender. A Nazi soldier walks over to the boy, draws his pistol, and shoots the boy in the chest.

"Noooo." A man's wail, pitched high as an animal's keen. The man appears. He lowers himself to the ground and cradles his dead son in his arms. The Nazi soldier comes up behind him, raises his pistol, and blows off the father's head.

The soldier faces the line of Jews. They are frozen, horrified, petrified. The Nazi soldier says simply, "If you want to live, keep moving."

Years later, my father will repeat those words to me.

"Ironic," he says. "The best piece of advice I ever got was from a pig of a Nazi soldier."

Many years later, as I lay in my hospital bed, my father's words will once again reverberate in my head: "Robert, if you want to live, you have to keep moving."

* * * * *

"What did you want to tell us, Daddy?"

Aliyah. Her eyes are wide blue moon circles.

I take her in and then I smile. "I just wanted to tell you that I love you very much. That's all. I don't feel so great right now. I'm really tired, but I'll see you later, okay?"

"You mean like in an hour?"

I move my eyes from Aliyah's to my father's and I fasten them there. "Yeah. Like in an hour."

"Let's go, kids. Let Daddy sleep." My dad breaks into a little half-jog, one of his hands squeezed around Aliyah's hand, the other enveloping Jacob's tiny hand like a catcher's mitt.

I watch them walk out of my room and then I turn my head toward the window.

The window.

I take a deep breath, close my eyes, and pray to God for sleep.

SESSION SEVEN

"FIGHTING BACK"

LOVE STORY

After my dad brings Aliyah and Jacob into my room and asks me to tell them that I've decided to jump out the window to my death, things start happening fast.

First and foremost, I commit to staying alive.

Which is not easy with cancer-killing poison coursing through my body, my face eternally hovering an inch above the toilet bowl, and my body feeling either as cold as Antarctica or as hot as the surface of the sun.

Not to mention the overall *pain.* Just picture yourself stepping out into the street and being hit by a car. *Wham.* And by a Hummer, not by a Mini Cooper.

Nope. It's not that easy staying alive.

But I'm not going anywhere. That's a fact. A certainty. I have now morphed into my dad. I am walking on my own miserable march, taking it step by painful step, teeny baby steps, some of them barely noticeable, but I'm always, *always* moving forward. I am going to make it. I am determined.

Slowly, moment by moment, hour by hour, day by day, I start to improve. Day three my fever fades and I can stand up unaided for a couple of minutes without keeling over from vertigo. Day four I can take a few steps without clutching my middle to quell the crippling nausea cramps.

By day seven, I'm able to sit up, focus on the TV, channel surf with the remote, and eventually lower myself out of bed and walk to the end of the room. A couple of days after that, my headache settles down to a low thrum, and I am, overall, fairly coherent.

Finally, Dr. Mehldau informs me that I can return home and gear up for my last chemo treatment. At last I can see the light at the end of the tunnel. I begin rooting myself on. *One more treatment. Just one more. You can do it.*

But I have changed. Enormously, deeply, incontrovertibly. The change takes the form of a constant gnawing pain in my gut that now grips me and holds on as if it has claws. The change has me twisted in knots. I know what it is, but I am afraid to speak its name aloud.

I decide to write about it. My support group recently suggested taking a personal inventory of our lives as a way of getting in touch with what really and truly matters. When you're staring eyeball to eyeball with the Grim Reaper, you'd better feel as if you've dealt with the important stuff. What's the point of going to your doom with a bunch of loose ends or unfulfilled dreams lying around? When else am I going to deal with my change, if not now? What am I waiting for?

One afternoon before I return home, my mother sits in my hospital room knitting a shawl or wall-to-wall carpeting and I sit up in bed, my reporter's notebook propped open between my knees. I scratch a few random lines across the top of the first page and say to myself, *Okay. I'm going to take a personal inventory of all the really important things in my life, listed by priority. What and who is really worth it? Who counts? Which people in my life are indispensable?*

Number one. That's obvious. *Family.* I carefully print my children's names, starting with the oldest, Jessica, ending with Jacob, the youngest. Then I write down my parents, Otto and Betty.

And then, without thinking, as if a Ouija board is powering the pen, I spell out: "M-E-L-I-S-S-A."

Yeah.

Melissa.

Okay, there it is. Right there. In black and white.

Melissa.

The instant after I write her name, I know that she is my number one priority. I have to see her. It's not important. It's *necessary.* I have to see Melissa if I live, or if I'm going to die. Either way. *I have to see her.*

Because here's the change within me that I dare not name:

I'm in love with Melissa.

Well, okay, again, full disclosure.

It's not really a change.

The truth is, Melissa has dominated my thoughts and taken up permanent residence in my heart since the day I broke up with her. I cannot stop seeing her face, hearing her laugh, smelling her perfume, her shampoo . . .

I believe that part of the pain I feel every day is the pain of losing Melissa.

So *here* is the real change:

I have to see her and tell her how I feel.

See, that's what cancer does. It shakes you up, then sifts out all the unimportant crap and leaves you facing only the highest priorities. Sounds eerie, but it's really not. It's what we should be doing every day. It's how we should live our lives. It's how I vow to live mine from now on.

Okay. Simple. I'm gonna tell Melissa how I feel.

I put down my pen and rub the top of my head. I count two major roadblocks blocking my way.

One. I haven't spoken to Melissa for six months. She doesn't know where I am or that I'm sick. She probably has a boyfriend. Or she might even have a husband.

"Holy shit," I say aloud.

Two. I have cancer. I look like hell. I feel like crap. Forget about a future with Melissa. I might not have a future, period. She's young. She has her whole life ahead of her. Why would she want to spend it with me?

"What holy shit?" My mom, speaking with a knitting needle in her mouth. I start to climb out of bed. I groan as I lower my legs to the floor. "Robert, where are you going?"

"Ma, you know what I'm thinking?"

"God knows."

"I'm thinking I want to go for a ride."

"Now?"

"Yeah. It's a beautiful day."

"It's a hundred and seventeen and it's noon."

"Let's go for a ride. Come on. You can drive."

"No. Really? You can barely put your shoes on."

"That's why you should drive." I somehow make it to the closet and manage to pull the flimsy plywood doors open. "A hundred seventeen. I guess I could wear shorts."

My mother rolls up her knitting and stares at me. "Robert, are you all right?"

I turn to her and put my hands on my hips. "Actually, Ma, I've changed."

"Changed? How?"

"I'll tell you in the car."

How long will it take you to drive me to Los Angeles?

I'm buzzed, goofy from the remnants of my medication and my new insane game plan. But that's what I'm thinking as I start fumbling through the closet, sliding hangers, searching for a shirt that might remotely fit, something that won't make me look like I'm wearing a tarp.

●　●　●　●　●

My mother drives, hands squeezing the hell out of the steering wheel at two and four o'clock, eyes squinting with unshakable focus into the desert sun. We don't say much. Two reasons. One, I'm too weak to speak. Two, I'm trying to figure out what I'm going to say to Melissa.

I rehearse a couple of opening lines in my head. Nothing seems right. Everything seems canned and forced.

"Where are we going?" my mother asks. Across her forehead runs a gulley of sheer, brutal concentration.

It suddenly strikes me: *My mother driving me to L.A.? This is not a good idea.* I cough and throw this plan out the window. I go to Plan B. "I have to make a phone call," I say.

"Out here? You have a phone in your room. We had to drive thirty miles for you to make phone call?"

"You can't call long distance from my hospital room." This is the truth and I realize now that it was the plan all along. I pause and pretend to look at something outside my window. "I have to call Melissa."

"Melissa." My mother's voice is matter-of-fact, without judgment.

"Yeah. See, here's the thing." I cough again, then clear my throat. When I speak now, my voice is low and gravelly, as if I'm channeling Tom Waits. "Ma, I miss her."

"That's natural. It's been a while since you've seen her or even talked to her, no? And you two were close—"

"No. I *really* miss her."

My mother raises an eyebrow. Great thing about me and my mom. We have a kind of shorthand. I don't have to say much. She gets what I mean after a very few words and sometimes just after a look. She keeps her eyes locked on the road. She spots something ahead, a desert mirage. "Look. Arrowhead Outlet Mall. Neiman Marcus has a pay phone. I've used it."

"Damn." I pat my pockets, then remember that they're empty. "I don't have any change."

"You can use my calling card."

She guns the car, speeds up toward the mall. She swoons. "I love this place."

"I know. It's your idea of Disneyland."

To confirm and annoy, she begins humming the tune to "It's a Small World."

* * * * *

The phone rings once, twice, and then right before the third ring, Melissa says, "Hello?"

Her voice is just as I remember—soft and tentative, bordering on shy. It's the most beautiful, sensuous voice I've ever heard, and just hearing her say that one word *Hello* has me practically clawing my way through the phone.

"Hi," is all I say.

Melissa pauses long enough to make lunch, to write a letter, to go to the store and come back. It is an *endless* pause. A gaping crater of a pause. For a second I think she has gone away or passed out. And then finally she says, "Robert?"

"Yeah."

"I didn't—where are you?"

"Phoenix. At a pay phone."

I switch ears. I sit down on a bench outside the department store and suck down about five gallons of oxygen. I need to gather my thoughts and, honestly, I just want to hear her breathe.

"Robert, how are you?"

She knows. Somehow she knows. She must've heard about my cancer on Stern.

I say, "Well, you know, up and down. But the good news is I only have one more chemo treatment and—"

"Wait. *Chemo?*"

"Melissa, I have cancer."

"Robert, you—"

Her voice sails off. For what seems like forever I hear nothing, not her breathing, nothing. I panic. I've lost the connection. I've lost *her*.

"Melissa?"

"I'm here." Her voice is a tiny echo.

"I thought you knew," I say after another mother of a pause. "I don't know why I thought that. I just . . . I don't know."

"I didn't know."

"Well, so, yeah, that's the story. That's where I've been. At the Mayo Clinic here in Arizona. I haven't been on an island cruise on the Love Boat or anything, if that's what you were thinking."

"I wasn't thinking that," she says.

"I have one more treatment," I say.

"And then, what, you know, what happens?"

"Toss of the coin," I say, then add quickly, "but the doctors are optimistic. I feel good. And I look fantastic. Really buff. The chemotherapy agrees with me. I've put on weight. I'm up to one twenty, one twenty-five."

She actually laughs.

"I really do weigh about a hundred and twenty," I say.

Melissa doesn't speak, but now I can hear her breathing again. I close my eyes and imagine the mist from her breath brushing my face.

"I really miss you," I say.

It must be my imagination but I think I can hear her heartbeat. I hear *thump-thump-thaa-thump* and then I realize that it's not hers at all, but mine. I'm hearing my own heart. My pulse is pounding and my armpits are soaked, my head is flushed, and I hear myself blurt out everything that's been swirling through my head: "I've never stopped thinking about you. Ever. Not for a second. Every day, morning, night, no matter what I'm going through that day, all I can think about is you. I can't stop myself. I can't help myself. I don't know what to do. But I can't imagine getting my last treatment and living the rest of my life, no matter how long that is going to be, without ever seeing you again. It just can't be like that. It can't. I can't allow that to be. The thought that I'll never see you again is killing me."

Thump-thump-thaa-thump.

Her breath caresses the phone.

I'm gonna pass out. Right here. Right now. In this outlet mall in Phoenix with my mother sitting on a bench fifty feet away knitting like a maniac. I'm burning up. I must have a fever. My forehead is a swamp. My cheeks feel like ovens.

Melissa says nothing. But now her breathing comes faster, racehorse fast. A drumbeat tapping in my ears. I've gotten to her. My speech has moved her. That was close. I wasn't sure how it was going over. I spoke from the heart, true, but you never know. This is going well.

"Robert?"

"Yes, Melissa?"

"I'm seeing someone. You told me it was over," she says. "You said not to call you and that you were never going to call me. You kept telling me to move on."

"I did. I know I did. I meant it at the time. I didn't want you to have to deal with me sick."

She sighs. I sigh back. Sigh and response. Well, now I have to ask the big question.

"Are you two, you know—?"

"We've been going out three weeks, a month, something like that."

And then Melissa chuckles. Hard to pick up irony over the phone but that's what I hear. Irony.

"What are you laughing at?"

"The Schimmel Touch," she says. "Rears its ugly head once again."

"Do I really want to hear this?"

"We slept together last night for the first time. Last night. Get it?"

"Perfect," I say. "Why couldn't I have called yesterday, right?"

"Yep."

"Yeah, well, I have the answer. Yesterday I thought for sure I was going to die. If there was one day that I didn't think about you twenty-four-seven, it was yesterday. Yesterday I was just trying to live."

"And today?"

"Today I just want to see you." I swallow and stare at my feet. And then I whisper. The words barely escape my lips. "Melissa, I miss you so much."

"Oh, Robert," she says. "I miss you, too. I really do. Shit."

And then she starts to cry.

That's all I need to hear. I hang up the phone and run over to my mother. Well, I don't actually run. I waddle as fast as I can. My mother looks up from her knitting. "How did it go?"

"I'm going to L.A. You have to drive me to the airport."

"What? You weren't supposed to leave the hospital. You're not even supposed to be *here*."

"I know. Come on, Ma, we gotta move."

She doesn't budge. She shoves her hands into the mountain of unknitted yarn on her lap. "First you get me to break you out of the hospital. Now you want me to help you leave the *state*?"

"Ma, please. I have to see her."

She tilts her head, studies me from a new angle, as if from this perspective she'll see or hear something different. "You can't stay over. You have to come back tonight."

"I will. I promise. It's an hour flight. I'll be back before midnight."

My mother shakes her head and hauls herself up to her feet. "I'm your mother. I'll cover for you."

"Thanks, Ma."

I kiss her on the cheek and walk like a penguin toward the car.

• • • • •

When I get to L.A. it's raining.

It rains once a year in L.A. and I pick the day. The Schimmel Touch once again.

By the time I rent a car and inch through the parking lot called rush hour from the airport to Melissa's apartment in West Hollywood, it's almost seven o'clock. Miraculously, I find a parking space on the street a block from her building. I start to get out of the car, stop, check myself in the mirror. It's been six months since I've seen her. I want to make a good impression, want to make sure I look great.

Let's see. I weigh a hundred twenty-five pounds. I'm wearing clothes that are three sizes too big. I've got on a baseball cap because I'm completely bald. I have no eyebrows or eyelashes. I look like something out of the bar scene in *Star Wars*.

Melissa's gonna see me and melt.

Or scream and go running out of the apartment.

Nothing I can do about it. I look the way I look. If she can't handle it, the trip was worth it because I'll know how she really feels. I'll go back to Mayo heartbroken and miserable, but at least I'll *know.* And I'll be able to move on. Maybe.

The rain has tapered to a drizzle. I push the car door open and somehow manage to extricate myself from the seat belt and climb out of the car. I feel like I'm a hundred years old. Every inch of me creaks. I shiver violently. I'm freezing and afraid. I still don't know what I'm going to say to her after all this time. Maybe it's best to say nothing, let her take the lead. No. I'm the one who broke us up. I have to take the lead. I have to take responsibility. She didn't want to break up with me. I have to remember that.

I should probably start with an apology. That really is the right thing to do because it's true. I am sorry. So, yeah, I'll open with a sincere apology, and then—

I'm here. Standing in front of her building. I stop and look up at her apartment. She lives on the second floor. And then, as if she can somehow feel me on the sidewalk below, she appears in the window, framed there like she's posing for a photograph. She tosses back her hair. She's let it grow out a little. It's still golden, luminous, like her. I wave. She smiles. She's radiant, even more beautiful than I had allowed myself to remember.

But she's not looking at me. She's not smiling at me. She's looking off at something inside her apartment. And then a guy appears next to her. He's tall, full head of black wavy hair, and here's the best part, the punch line, he's shirtless. And his stomach muscles *ripple*. Forget a six-pack. He's got a twenty-four pack. A case. She's going out with the guy in the Calvin Klein underwear ad.

And now they're kissing. Melissa and Abs of Steel. Right up there, framed in the window. Then, of course, the topper, the rain kicks up. The intermittent trickle becomes a stabbing downpour. I stand on the sidewalk, two floors down, pelted by the rain, watching Melissa kissing the shirtless male model and I realize that things are not going as well as I'd hoped.

I'm frozen. The rain is dripping down off the bill of my cap, drenching my shirt, and I can't move. Do I yell up at her? Do I throw rocks at her window? Do I knock on her door? Do I drive back to the airport and hop on the first plane back to Phoenix?

Jesus. They're still kissing.

Have a heart. Or at least close the shades.

I slosh and stumble back to the car. In the blinding rain, rented windshield wipers slapping feebly at the wet arrows soaking the glass, I creep across Beverly Boulevard and end up back in my apartment, a one-bedroom in Hollywood that I lease still, for no apparent reason. No reason until now, when it has become my safe haven. Shelter from the storm.

I wring myself out in the living room, pace, trying to think. What's my next move? Do I even have a next move? Is this hopeless? Crazy? Stupid? Probably all three.

But I heard her voice a few hours ago. I heard her cry. I felt what she was feeling and I know, I just *know* that she's feeling exactly the same way that I'm feeling. Which is why I'm here. And, cancer lesson seven, I'm not giving up.

I'm strangely calm. I'm not even upset that she's kissing the Calvin Klein underwear guy. She has every right. I broke up with her. She moved on. She doesn't know I'm here.

I have to tell her. I have to get to her.

I pick up my pace. I walk from room to room, living room, bedroom, kitchen, dinette, thinking, hoping to find some clue somewhere—

And then I see it.

On the nightstand.

The Worst-Case Scenario Survival Guide.

The book Melissa gave me last year for my birthday.

Talk about irony. I'm *living* the worst-case scenario right now. I've got cancer, I've fled the hospital in Phoenix to return to the arms of the love of my life, only to find her standing in the window kissing Stan Studmuffin.

I pick up the book and turn to the first page. A year ago Melissa had signed it and written, "There'll never be a worst case scenario because I love you forever and there will never be anyone for you but me."

I rip out the page.

I stuff it into my pocket and head back outside to the car, which I'd parked illegally in a red zone, figuring there's no way the parking police are writing tickets in this weather. Wrong. Flapping under my windshield like a trapped duck is a $125 ticket, soaked and half-shredded. I crumple it up and toss it onto the passenger seat. At some point, my luck's gotta change, right? Yeah. After fifty years of the Schimmel Touch, tonight's the night. What are the chances of that?

Squinting through the driving rain, I creep back to Melissa's apartment building. Head swiveling, casing the area as if I'm a thief, I pull into her parking garage. I spot her car. My heart's racing as I get out of the rental car and stick the page of *The Worst-Case Scenario Survival Guide*, the page on which she's promised her undying love in *writing*, under her windshield wipers. I pat the page, hustle back into the car, and drive the hell out of there as fast as I dare. As I skid out of her garage, I blink. The rain has stopped and the sky, with the sun sinking, has become a brilliant shade of red and gold. This sudden whipsaw change in the weather doesn't mean anything, does it? It's not a sign that my luck is finally turning around, is it? Nah. Just coincidence.

Now, back to my apartment for the second part of my ingenious plan, which is—

Well, okay, there is no second part. There really wasn't a first part. So now I wait. And pace some more. Maybe I'll throw in a little praying. Then I might try some visualization. Add a dash of positive thinking.

Ah, shit. Melissa might not even see the page. Or she might see it and toss it in the trash.

This was a horrible idea. A desperate move by a desperate man. A wild shot in the dark. I should drive back to her apartment and pull the page off her car. I crash through the living room and wrestle my sweatshirt back on. I reach for the door handle and—

The phone rings.

I stare at it.

It really did ring. Right? I want to be sure.

It rings again.

I let it ring a third time. Can't appear too anxious. Have to play this cool even though my heart has flown into my throat and feels like it's gonna hop right out of my mouth.

Fourth ring.

I'm all over the phone.

I fling it up against my ear, drop it, catch it, cradle it between my cheek and shoulder and I speak, trying to sound nonchalant, casual, even slightly annoyed as if I expect the caller to be a solicitor.

"Hello?"

"So you're in town, huh?"

"Yeah." I switch ears because the receiver is soaked in my sweat. "How did you know?"

"Take a guess."

"You found the note."

"Actually, no, I didn't," Melissa says. "The guy I'm seeing went to get us something to eat and *he* found it."

"Oh. Shit."

"Yeah. He came back upstairs and said, 'What the fuck is this?'"

"Awkward."

"A little bit." She holds a beat. "It's not important."

Another beat. Longer. Now my heart feels lodged in my throat like a brick.

"I want to see you," Melissa says.

"I don't want to force you into anything because if you and he are serious—"

"Robert, I want to see you."

Now I hold, but just long enough to blink away the tears that are welling up. "I want to see you, too, Melissa," I croak out.

"I'm coming over."

"Well, the thing is, when you see me, you might be—"

Click. The dial tone hums and then howls for what seems forever and I can't stop it because I'm nailed to the floor. And then there is a soft knock on the door five minutes later, maybe ten, I can't be sure, but I open the door and there she is, Melissa, and she looks at me without judgment, she looks at me with simple *longing,* and then we're holding on to each other and our tears are flowing and we can't tell whose are whose because our faces are pressed together.

"I've always loved you," she murmurs. "Always. I never stopped."

"What about your, you know, friend?"

"As soon as I read the note, I told him it was over."

"Just like that?"

She shrugs. "Kind of. I told him my boyfriend was back."

"Back from the dead," I say.

She lets out a moan, a sob, and she holds me tighter, and I hold her with all my might, which isn't much, and I know I have to get back to Mayo and get through my last treatment, but this moment and what I have now with Melissa I know is forever, and then I'm crying because I know I will never let her go again, not ever.

And then as I kiss her and she grazes my cheeks and lips with tiny sweet kisses, I can't help but wonder where I'd be if Calvin the Underwear King had half a brain and had ripped up the note and thrown it away.

SESSION EIGHT

"GETTING STUNG"

DECEMBER 12, 2000

So I'm sitting in a chair in Dr. Mehldau's office, at Mayo, waiting for the results.

I've just undergone a battery of tests and I'm still in my hospital gown. I scan the room. There's my mom, sitting across from me, her mouth clamped tight into a razor-thin line. There's my dad at the window, hands clasped behind his back, staring at I don't know what and neither does he.

We wait in silence. The air is thick, clogged with tension and nerves. It's been six months since I first got the news. Doesn't feel like it. Feels more like six years.

"Where is he?" my dad asks, his patience shot. "What, did he get a better offer?"

My mom touches him lightly on the forearm. "Otto, he's a busy man. He'll be here."

My dad shrugs. Unclasps his hands. Pats down his pants pockets as if he's lost his money clip.

Six months.

That's how long I've known cancer. And Dr. Mehldau.

Feels as if I've known him forever. Feels like he's part of my family. Maybe because from day one he's taken me in like a long-lost brother. At his urging, I've never hesitated to call him anytime, day or night, when I've felt panicked or alone. He's my teacher, my cancer mentor, my Yoda, my Dr. Phil. He pushes when I need a shove, puts an arm around me when I need encouragement. I love him.

It must be really difficult for doctors to become personally involved with their patients. I don't see how they do it. There's too much risk. So many patients don't make it. I don't know how they deal with the constant loss. Let's face it, doctors are just regular people. They're not miracle workers. They're not special human beings who've been touched by God.

That's something I've never understood. Why do most people put doctors on such a pedestal? People do that with certain professions. Like pilots. *Wow. He's a pilot. You gotta be a special kind of person to be a pilot.*

Yeah. A person who passes a flying test.

I might actually go too far the other way when I think of doctors. I think they're completely normal, shmoes like the rest of us. Which is why I worry. I worry that my guy is at a party getting shit-faced and all of a sudden his beeper goes off, he goes to the phone and hears, "You gotta get down here right away. We're doing Schimmel's kidney transplant right now." Even if he's had four glasses of wine, I don't think he'll ever say, "Yeah, you know what? I ain't gonna make it."

Nope. He starts shooting back cups of black coffee, and half in the bag or not, he's at the hospital scrubbing up, about to open me up for the kidney transplant.

I find it amusing that people put so much trust in doctors. They'll do anything they say. If their doctor says, "Okay, now we're gonna stick this thing up your ass," most people say, "Whatever you think," no questions asked.

I'm gonna ask a few questions. I'm gonna ask other people and find out if they've ever had that particular procedure done.

He wanted to stick what up your ass? He was probably drunk.

I'm thinking about this and smiling while Dr. Mehldau slips into the room undetected. He grins back. "What's so funny?"

"I was just thinking about you and I started to laugh."

"Not that many people find their oncologists amusing," he says.

"I see humor in a lot of weird shit," I say.

"I've noticed," he says. He suddenly claps his hands, which scares the crap out of both of us. "Okay. I've got good news and bad news. First the good news. Your tests came back clean. As of today, you are officially in remission."

For a moment, I feel nothing, then I feel numb. I start to speak, can't. Then I finally manage: "You mean, I'm . . . *cured?*"

"I don't like to use that word," Dr. Mehldau says. "I prefer *remission*. Remission means that you are asymptomatic and that there's no sign of cancer at this time. You can expect two to three years cancer-free. Some doctors might push that out to three to five years."

"And then?" my mom asks.

"We take it year by year," Dr. Mehldau says.

"Day by day," my dad says, lowering the bar. "Like life."

"Your dad's right," Dr. Mehldau says. "That's how we really have to look at it. Day to day."

"Cancer-free," I say, trying it on.

"Doesn't mean that you're cured," Dr. Mehldau says.

"Don't worry," my mom says, dabbing a clump of Kleenex at her makeup that's pooled up because of her tears. "He's cured."

"Remission," I say. "I'm trying to cry but you've been beating the shit out of me for six months and I got no crying left."

"You're not out of the woods," Dr. Mehldau says. "You will still have to undergo blood tests, PET scans, and CAT scans every couple of months for a year. Then every four months or so, then six months, and so on. It's nothing out of the ordinary. Just part of the deal. You'll have to adjust to that."

"Beats the alternative," I say.

"By a mile," Dr. Mehldau says.

"Yeah," I say. Then the dam bursts and we're all crying— my mom and I quietly, my dad coughing like a thunderclap to cover his sobs. I even catch Dr. Mehldau wiping at his nose. Suddenly I remember to ask him: "What's the bad news?"

Dr. Mehldau lights up. "See that nurse out there? I'm not screwing her."

I hop off the table and throw my arms around Dr. Mehldau and hug him. He hugs me back and then I give him a long wet kiss on the cheek. I don't give a shit that my hospital gown is riding up my ass. For all I care, he can grab both my butt cheeks and knead them like he's making a *challah*.

●　●　●　●　●

I sit in the green room at the Monte Carlo in Las Vegas. I'm about to perform onstage for the first time since I've been diagnosed. I'm surprisingly relaxed. My parents and Lee, my manager, sit squished on the couch with me, a crazy family portrait. Adam, the Monte Carlo's PR guy, sits opposite us in an armchair. He's fidgety as hell. I've known Adam for years.

"What are you gonna open with?" Adam asks.

I catch Lee's eye. "The cancer," I say. "I'm gonna talk about that."

Lee nods. "You have to be true to yourself."

Adam's mouth twitches. "The cancer? I don't know."

"Well, that's what I'm gonna do," I say. I'm not combative. I'm just stating a fact.

Adam says, "Robert, the audience doesn't want to hear about your cancer. It's not funny."

"You're right. Cancer's not funny. But how I dealt with it is."

"Those slides? I don't know." Adam gets up, pours himself some coffee. He shakes his head. "I can't believe you're even here. You should've canceled."

"Adam," I say patiently. "I have to get back onstage. I have to prove to myself that I can still do it."

Suddenly I stop.

"You know what?" I say. "That's not true. I know I can still make people laugh. But this is no longer about that. It's not even about me. I'm speaking for a lot of other people now. I *have* to talk about the cancer."

"It just makes me uncomfortable, Robert."

"Look at me."

Adam keeps his eyes down, avoiding mine. He distracts himself by stirring two packets of artificial sweetener into his coffee.

"Look at me."

I pull myself to my feet. I tip the scales now at a sleek 128 pounds. I still have no hair. Not a strand anywhere on my body. Still no eyebrows or eyelashes. Not even ear fuzz. My cheeks are sunken. My skin is the color of chalk.

"What am I gonna do," I say quietly, facing him, "tell jokes about bad airplane food?"

Adam says nothing. He rips open another packet of the sweetener and stirs it into the coffee.

"The audience knows what's going on," I say. "They've heard me on Stern. Or if they haven't and I walk out looking like this, they're going to say, 'What happened to that guy?' I can't ignore my fucking *life*."

Adam. Still stirring his coffee. Thinking. He's a good guy. Suddenly the expression on his face shifts and I can tell that he knows that I'm asking him to fight with me.

"Don't have much choice, do I?" he says.

The door opens and the stage manager motions to me.

"This is it," I say.

My parents climb to their feet. My dad circles his arms around me.

"Keep moving," he whispers.

My mother cups my face in her hands. "I love you," she says and kisses me.

Lee pats me on the back. "I really admire you, Robert," he says.

I smile and start toward the door.

"Robert," Adam says, insistent, stopping me.

"Yeah?"

"Knock 'em dead." Adam offers up his fist. I fist him back. Two fifty-year-old white guys playing ghetto.

"Speaking of death," I say, pointing at his coffee. "That shit'll kill you."

To the echo of *ROBERTTTT SCHIMMELLL* booming through the sound system, I step onto the stage. My phantom body tiptoes to the center illuminated by the spotlight's orange glow. My black suit hangs off me, ridiculously oversized, as if I've pulled something out of Schwarzenegger's closet. I wave at the crowd and then, as one, they are on their feet, howling, clapping, stomping, and tears stream down my face. This is a first. I've never had a standing ovation *before* I've spoken a word. I blow a kiss back at them and I tell them my story, the story of the last seven months of my life, of how Dr. Mehldau told me I had non-Hodgkin's lymphoma, and how I went through chemotherapy and licked the Big C. I tell them jokes about the dick wig salesman, and sitting next to Bill and wanting to bang Nadine the chemo nurse (all of whom are in the audience). At the end of my set, I click through a dozen slides, showing me in the hospital at my absolute weakest point. I look gaunt and withered but I'm laughing. I pepper the slides with jokes. The audience howls, laughing louder here than at any of my earlier sex jokes. Finally, I tell them that all of this, all of *them,* has been my inspiration and that this game ain't over, not by a long shot. It is only just beginning.

They are on their feet again, applauding, whistling, and some of them are crying. I wait for them to sit back down and I tell them how wonderful they've been and how incredible I feel, thanks to them. And then I hit them with the topper.

"There's somebody I want you to meet," I say. "The guy who got me through this."

I point to the third row and introduce Dr. Mehldau. The audience applauds, then as I urge them on, they roar. Dr. Mehldau reluctantly stands up and offers the crowd a tentative finger waggle. Before he can sit back down, I ask him to join me onstage. He doesn't want to, but with the audience now cheering wildly, refusing to take no for an answer, he sidesteps out of his row and comes onstage. We hug and the audience claps again.

I explain how with cancer, you're never cured. I explain about how my life will now consist of a nonstop regimen of tests. But mainly I talk about how cancer has changed my life.

"I'm thankful to be alive. You have no idea," I say. "Tonight I feel privileged to have been able to give you a small gift, the gift of laughter." I then lay a hand on Dr. Mehldau's shoulder. "Dr. Mehldau has given me the greatest gift of all. He's given me the gift of time."

The audience applauds.

"He's given me more time on earth, more time with my family, more time with my loved ones, and he's taught me how to appreciate every moment I have. Precious time."

More applause. Then I face Dr. Mehldau. "Dr. Mehldau, there's no way I can ever repay you, but here is a small token of thanks for giving me this gift of time."

I drop my hand from his shoulder, reach into my pocket, and pull out a watch, still in its case.

"Thank you, Dr. Mehldau," I say, presenting him with the watch.

Wild applause.

Now he's actually crying. Finally, he pulls himself together and says, "It's beautiful. I don't know how to thank you."

"By coming up onstage tonight, you just did. I just hope that once in a while, when you look at your watch, you'll think of me. That way you won't forget me. Because I know I will never forget you."

The audience goes nuts.

LESSONS

So that's it. How my life changed for the better because of cancer. Somehow the eight chemo sessions taught me these simple, yet profound life lessons:

Keep your sense of humor, no matter what.
Create a purpose, a focus, and never take your eyes off it.
Figure out what's important to you. What's really important.
Be open. Try anything. You never know.
Love. You need love. Tons of it. A shitload of love.
Sometimes you need to be selfish.
You need support. You're in this alone, but you can't fight it alone.
The most precious thing you have is time. Don't waste it.

You're only human.
And, finally, once again—
Laugh.

THE GODFATHER

You might also say that cancer settled things between Vicki and me and brought Melissa and me together. Melissa and I talk about that. Sometimes I think we were just destined to be together, no matter what. I know this. Once we were a couple, we wanted to share everything in our lives, including children. Unfortunately, the doctors said that was out of the question. Even my biggest supporter, Dr. Mehldau, said it was never gonna happen. I was fifty-three, had one ball, and had undergone six months of intensive chemotherapy, which certainly zapped any fertility I had left in me.

Guess what? The doctors were wrong.

On June 5, 2003, three years to the *day* that I was diagnosed with non-Hodgkin's lymphoma, we had a son.

In the hospital that day after holding Sam, then bathing him, and laying him on top of Melissa for his first feeding, I called Dr. Mehldau and asked him if he wanted to be the godfather of the kid he said I'd never have. He said he'd be delighted.

Melissa and I didn't stop there. Two years later, our son Max was born. I was fifty-five, still one-balled, and still, thank God, bless Jesus, praise Allah, and love you, Buddha, cancer-free.

MARCH 2007

A late afternoon. Melissa, Sam, Max, and I are at the beach. They sit on the blanket. I walk along the shore. I toss pebbles into the ocean and sniff the salt air. Miniscule waves break softly over my bare feet.

The sun begins to set. I wave to Melissa and the kids. The kids race toward me. Melissa follows a few feet behind.

"Look at that," I say. "Just look at that sunset."

It's a Technicolor masterpiece, a brilliant God painting. Neon oranges, blues, violets. We walk slowly, basking in the sunset. My hands encircle my sons' tiny hands. Random squawks from distant seagulls and the whoosh from the waves are the only sounds. The colors from the sunset pour down on us, bathe us.

"This is unbelievable," I say. "This is Paradise. It really is."

Melissa smiles, rests her head on my shoulder. There could not be a more perfect moment.

I plant one foot in the sand and step on a bee.

I scream at the top of my lungs. *"MOTHERFUCKER-SONOFAFUCKINGSHITTT!!!"*

I drop my sons' hands and hop around, the bee sting cutting through my foot like a knife.

"SHIIIITTTTT! I stepped on a fucking bee!"

"Don't scream like that!" Melissa screams. "You're scaring the kids!"

I glance at Sam and Max. They're staring at me, not sure whether to laugh or cry.

"Shit!" I howl. "My foot!"

"Robert, stop it! We don't want them to be afraid of bees," Melissa says. "Daddy's just playing."

"I am not! Mother*fucker*!"

I plop down on the sand and pull my foot toward me so that I can examine the bottom. A two-inch bee stinger protrudes from the middle of my foot, poking up like a tiny flagpole. I grab it and yank it out.

I look at the collective faces of my family. Melissa's, frowning, horrified, pissed; Max's, stunned, scared; and Sam's, vaguely amused. I shake my head and laugh.

"I'm okay," I say. "I just stepped on a bee. It's fine. No big deal. I have another foot."

"Let's help Daddy up," Melissa says.

My family surrounds me. Melissa and Sam grab my hands and Max pushes me from behind and then I'm on my feet, walking slowly, limping slightly, dull pain throbbing along the bottom of my foot.

"I'll live," I say. "Scared the shit out of me, though."

"Really?" Melissa says, and laughs. I tickle Sam and Max and now they're giggling and running ahead of us. I drape an arm across Melissa's shoulder and she weaves her fingers through mine. Clinging to each other, we walk along the shore as the sun starts to dip down below the horizon.

Well, there it is. The key to life in a nutshell:

Life is good. It really is.

But sometimes you get stung.

Some people who get stung on the beach will never go back. Before cancer, I might have been one of those people. I might've packed up my family and gotten the hell out of there. Getting stung would've ruined the rest of the day. No more. You have to learn to bounce back. Otherwise you could miss a beautiful sunset.

Life ain't about the bee.

It's about the beach.

ACKNOWLEDGMENTS

ROBERT:

There are so many people I would like to thank. I'm certain that I could fill a book with just those names. But in the midst of global warming, and the spirit of green living, I've limited myself to a pretty short list. So, if you aren't mentioned, do not take it personally. Instead, find solace in the fact that you're helping to save a tree and protect the environment.

My beautiful children: Jessica, Aliyah, Derek, Jacob, Sam, and Max. You all always bring so much laughter, joy, and love into my life.

My wife, Melissa, who appeared in my life just at the right moment and turned it upside down. There hasn't been a day that goes by that you are not in my every heartbeat.

To Mom and Dad. For your unconditional love and support. And for getting me through the darkest days of my life by helping me see the light.

My sister, Sandy, for her faith and love. She believed in me even before I did. It is because of her that I got onstage the first time. Otherwise, I'd be a fifty-seven-year-old stereo salesman today.

My brother, Jeffrey, for his love, passion for perfection, and always doing everything in his power to protect me. In 1992, Jeff was my writing partner on *In Living Color*. In reality, Jeff did all of the writing.

Special thanks to Lee Kernis. The man who hid my kids at his house while I was on the lam. My personal manager. My friend. A real genuine guy. There will never be anyone like him again.

Thanks to Rick Greenstein and everyone at the Gersh Agency.

Thanks to everyone at Da Capo Press, especially Ben Schafer, Marnie Cochran, Renee Caputo, and Donna Moore. And David Vigliano and Kirby Kim of Vigliano and Associates.

Thanks to Keenan, Damon, Shawn, and Marlon Wayans for their support. I owe my last visit with my son to Keenan.

Thank you Lance Burton, Nivea Santiago, and the staff of the Monte Carlo for gambling on me by letting me onstage while I was still going through treatment.

Thanks to Howard Stern for all his support. He personally called me while I was in the hospital getting chemotherapy and asked if I thought I'd make it to New Year's Eve. Because he had me in the death pool, and Robin had Anthony Quinn.

Bob and Tom, Lamont Tonelli, and all of the radio show hosts who called and kept me alive with my fans by putting me on the air during my hospital visits.

Tom Cruise. He visited my son Derek at Children's Hospital during the filming of *Days of Thunder*. There was no entourage with him. No publicist. No paparazzi. Just Tom. Just him spending time with my little boy. Thanks, Tom.

Carey Strom, M.D. For his heartfelt advice and friendship. He's the only guy I'd feel comfortable giving me a colonoscopy in the privacy of his home.

Thanks to Vicki for taking such loving care of our son Derek. You devoted your entire life to him during his illness. You were not only his mother, but also his hospice nurse and advocate. Thank you for being understanding and for giving me the opportunity to spend quality time with my children while I was sick, and helping me get through my treatment.

Jay Leno, for his support when Derek was in the hospital.

Jerry Lewis, the man who inspired me to become a comedian in the first place.

Also a special thanks to William E. McEuen, Bob Merlis, Jeff Gold, Russ Thyret, Martin Landau, Steve Martin, Alan Metter, Mike Scully, Ronnie Weinstein, Jay Rosenthal, Theodore Braich, M.D., John Camoriano, M.D., David Mulligan, M.D., David Douglas, M.D., Marc Golden, Michael Gendler, Jeff Glieberman, Penny Salomon, Rick Murdock, Budd Friedman, Ira Kurgan, Sandy Grushow, Dr. Peter Sheerin, Eric Gold, Rodney Dangerfield, Jerry Lewis, Robert Hartman, Dan Mer, Bill Blumenreich, Tim Sarkes, Billy Crystal, Conan O'Brien, and Mel Gibson.

Very special thanks to Alan Eisenstock. Without him, this book would not exist. Alan and I had a special bond right from the beginning. I learned that he also suffered the loss of a child. His son Zachary. I knew then that if there were anyone that could help me express my true feelings, he'd be the one. And he did. During our sessions together we both shared a lot of tears. Some from laughter. Some from memories. His passion for helping me tell my story in my words was never-ending. (Although a lot of the F-words were mysteriously taken out.)

And God. Who, after taking my only son, graced me threefold with three more sons in return. I am truly blessed!

ALAN:

Thank you, Robert, for your courage, your spirit, your passion, and for making me laugh longer and harder than anyone else ever has. You are an inspiration.

Thank you, Melissa, for being Robert's rock, our driver, the mother of the year, the voice of reason, the keeper of the kingdom.

Thanks to David Vigliano, Kirby Kim, and Michael Harriot.

Thanks to everyone at Da Capo Press, especially Ben Schafer, Marnie Cochran, and Renee Caputo.

Thank you, David Ritz.

Thanks to Shirley and Jim Eisenstock; Madeline and Phil Schwarzman; Susan Pomerantz and George Weinberger; Susan Baskin and Richard Gerwitz; Loretta, Brian, Linda, Lorraine, Diane, Alan, Chris, Ben, and Nathan; Art Goldman; Edwin Greenberg and Elaine Gordon; Linda Nussbaum; Bruce and Judy Levitt; Linda Bowen; Kathy

Montgomery and Jeff Chester; Randy Turtle; Randy Feldman; David Goodman and Wendy Felson; David Perren; Joyce Barkin; Diane Golden; Judi Farkas; Bob Vickrey; Tony Koursaris of Taverna Tony in Malibu, our office; and Katie O'Laughlin and her incredible staff at Village Books in Pacific Palisades, my hangout.

Thanks always to the Miracles—Bobbie, Jonah, and Kiva.

Finally, thanks to my constant companion, Snickers the Wonder Dog, who loves everything I write and laughs at everything I say. At least I think she does.

Authors' Note: Dr. "Mehldau" is actually a compilation of several doctors who treated Robert over the course of his diagnosis and chemotherapy.